Where's My Pen?

A Guide to Supporting People With Dyspraxia

Sarah Johns

chipmunkapublishing
the mental health publisher
empowering people with dyspraxia

Sarah Johns

All rights reserved, no part of this publication may be reproduced by any means, electronic, mechanical photocopying, documentary, film or in any other format without prior written permission of the publisher.

> Published by
> Chipmunkapublishing
> PO Box 6872
> Brentwood
> Essex CM13 1ZT
> United Kingdom

http://www.chipmunkapublishing.com

Copyright © Sarah Johns 2009

Chipmunkapublishing gratefully acknowledges the support of Arts Council England.

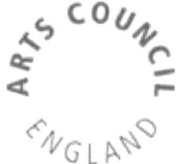

Where's My Pen?

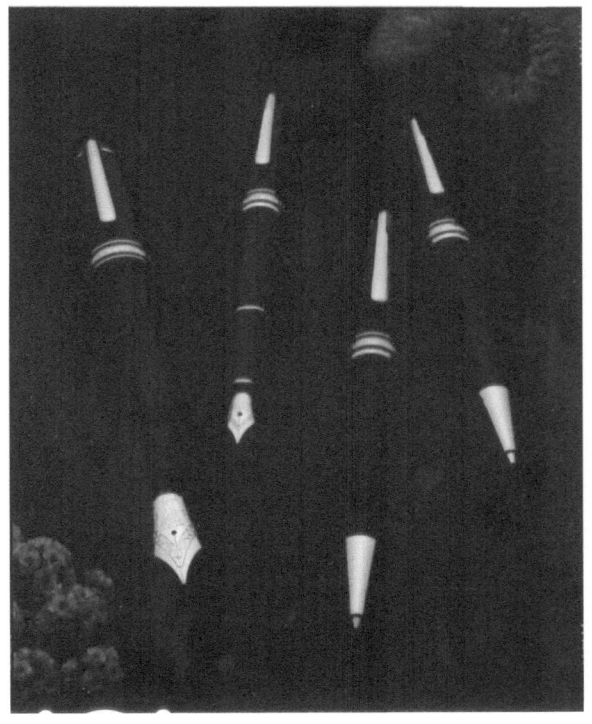

Photograph by Sean Hoyland

Sarah Johns

Where's My Pen?

Disclaimer:

I am not claiming to be an expert on dyspraxia nor am I hoping to review literature involving the citation of authors. I am doing this to raise awareness about dyspraxia. The experiences have come from my own personal situations and for confidential reasons I have not included names apart from in the acknowledgements. The advice given is from me and I would advise people to consult an expert for further diagnosis and/or support for dyspraxia.

There may be some sections where the language might be hard to understand. This is a challenge for me and often it can be difficult to be succinct when explaining something. Please bear with me.

Best wishes,

Sarah

Sarah Johns

Where's My Pen?

Acknowledgements

I would like to thank all my family, Olly and all my friends for the support they have given me through tough times and good times. I could not and would not be here if it wasn't for you all.

Thank you to PJ Hughes who helped to find me a publisher for this book and also to Amy Clarke for designing an amazing front cover. Thank you to Sean for the photographs of the pens! I really appreciate all your help. Special thanks to Chipmunka, the publishers, for producing this book!

Thank you to Alison who has been really supportive, it has meant such a lot to me and also to people at work, especially Angie, for being so patient.

Thanks to Lorraine who has been very supportive and introduced me to a really effective treatment which I have written about. It has really helped me in all aspects of my life.

Thanks to all the people I have worked with and hope to work with in the future. I am genuinely interested in learning/developmental difficulties and fascinated by the many people I have met with amazing personalities. Everyone has something to offer, so don't ever give up!

Sarah Johns

Where's My Pen?

Introduction

I keep pinching myself every time I think that I have written a book as it is such an achievement for me. I have always thought of having a go at writing but have attempted it, written half a page and then bizarrely found the washing up very enjoyable for the first time ever. With this book, I have written about something I am really passionate about and when that happens I don't think it becomes a chore or an effort. This experience has provided me with a chance to offer support and guidance about a condition called dyspraxia with the aim of raising awareness about the learning difficulty/difference (LD). The reasons why I have written this book will unfold as you read through and hopefully you will learn something new and read with interest.

It is amazing how many people have said to me, "dyspraxia, ooh what's that? I've heard of dyslexia but not dyspraxia". From my experiences so far, I feel this can often be a hidden condition. I have had many people who know me, saying, "How can you be dyspraxic when you have done a degree?" By the end of this book hopefully aspects of the condition will become clearer and it may help increase people's understanding about it. From talking about some of the challenges I have faced, I am not on a quest for sympathy, I just hope to demonstrate some of the symptoms of dyspraxia and how they manifest themselves in different forms.

As the title of this book suggests, it will hopefully help people of any age and walks of life, demonstrating some real life situations where dyspraxia could present itself. One thing to remember is that people suffering from the condition can present strengths and challenges in different ways. However, at the same time, there are common symptoms which tend to occur within the condition. I just hope from writing this book, it will help people use some of the suggestions or it will spark off a parent or friend/sufferer to come up with their own ways of supporting someone with dyspraxia. I really hope this is useful, which is the main reason for me writing this!

There are lots of reasons why I wanted to write this book and believe me a few times I thought, should I do it, should I not? In the end I thought, what is the worst that could happen? Here goes….

Where's My Pen?

Chapter One: How This Book Came About

This chapter aims to demonstrate how this book came about and includes a brief overview of certain aspects of my life. I am thirty years old at the time of writing and do not have an official diagnosis of dyspraxia yet but am in the process of finding out how to get an assessment. Already, it has been a challenge as the condition can often be detected more so during childhood than adulthood. However, I think the reason it was not detected when I was a child was because there was not as much awareness about the condition as there is today. I am hoping the awareness will continue to increase over the next few years and people will understand more and more about LDs.

In my quest for an answer to explain why I found certain aspects of my life a challenge, I came across dyspraxia. I know a lot of people can become paranoid and think they have various ailments and conditions, but after researching a lot into this condition, I realised a lot of my experiences from past and present pointed towards this LD.

The time in my life when I feel dyspraxia affected my health the most, was during my study at university and the first few years of work. I went straight from school to study for a sports degree in Cardiff and then a few years later, I went onto study for a physiotherapy degree. When I began working as a physiotherapist it was then that the possible dyspraxic symptoms came more apparent. I was working in a very busy environment and had to think on my feet on several occasions. This is hard for anyone when under pressure, but I felt like my brain was struggling to process all the information I needed and my coping mechanisms were not helping me. To show you an example, if I had to treat patients on a hospital ward, I knew what had to be done and could probably tell people the sensible plan, but when it came to putting it into practice, it was hard to sequence everything. Too much information was feeding into my mind at once and so it felt like lots of scrambled information was circulating around in my head which wasn't helpful to me or anyone.

As you could imagine, this made me feel extremely stressed and as a result I went into a severe depression, something which is explored further in this book. This wasn't to say that I was dangerous in my practice as I was aware of my difficulties, but it meant I was slower with my work. The times when I was worrying were the times I should have been focussing on aspects of my work, so this affected my thought processes. Eventually, I had become so stressed with everything, I couldn't cope anymore and it's amazing how the body has a funny way of saying enough is enough. I had to take time out of physiotherapy and recover from the depression and whilst I was off work, I came across an exercise programme which focussed on part of the brain called the cerebellum. The aim was to help relieve symptoms of LDs. Although this did not cure me, it genuinely did help me a lot and I am about to take my driving test, something I never

Where's My Pen?

thought I would actually feel comfortable with. I ended up working for the company and really enjoyed working within this field of work and had a lot of empathy for children and adults with a LD. Unfortunately the company went into financial difficulties and I was made redundant. I wanted to stay within the same line of work so at the time of writing this book, I have a job working for a charity, which supports adults with Aspergers/autism, another very interesting condition. Within the charity, there are also a few people we support who have Aspergers and dyspraxia, so this has been really interesting for me. Because of my experiences, I have a general knowledge and genuine interest about LDs. As a result, I have worked with children and adults with varying talents and abilities. I have tried to return to physiotherapy but unfortunately it has become harder to gain employment within this field at present. My ideal job would be to combine all my skills and experience to treat a person with a LD in a holistic way.

One of my aims in writing this book is to educate people so dyspraxia can continue to be detected earlier in life. If it had been picked up earlier with me, perhaps I would not have experienced the depression in later life. At the same time, I am not blaming anyone or anything for my situation as I do think if these experiences had not happened, I would not have written this book. However, I would like to help people avoid going through the depression and stress that I had to experience for nearly two years.

There are positive aspects of going through a tough patch in life, even though it doesn't seem like it at the time. It really does make you stronger as a person and appreciate things that can often be taken for granted. I do not worry about silly things now and what people think of me. I have had support from my difficulties beyond belief in the form of my close friends and family but have also had negative attitudes in other situations including past employment. A word of advice to anyone involved with a LD is to stay true to yourself as there will always be people who do not understand LDs and will say the classic line of "you are just using it as an excuse". I hope you take something from this book, even if it means you get an idea of how to support someone with dyspraxia or it makes you appreciate what skills and positive attributes you have to offer if you suffer from a LD.

Sit back, relax, eat that chocolate bar or apple (balanced diet of course!) and enjoy the book. I have not made this book too long as I always found it hard to sustain a long book and was put off by it before I even began reading. I also hope you find the print outs helpful if it is an e-book or the advice pages if you are reading the paperback. I have tried to compile advice and support that you can realistically try, so best of luck-never give up!

Where's My Pen?

Chapter Two: An Introduction To Dyspraxia

Have a think of how much you know about LDs and then think back to how much you were taught at school. I could imagine that not everyone reading this will have been educated at school about Dyslexia, Dyspraxia, Attention Deficit Hyperactivity Disorder or Asperger Syndrome/Autism. If you are reading this thinking, "well actually I know loads about them", is that because you have learnt about it at a later age or is it from school? The only reason I say this is because I don't feel enough awareness is taught in schools about different LDs. I know it may not be a priority over English, maths and science but I do feel people should be more aware of the conditions out there. There seems to be more awareness than previous years but there still needs to be even more. There can sometimes be a misconception that someone with a LD is not very intelligent, but often people are of average or above average intelligence and may just learn in different ways. Sometimes if people know you have a LD they may talk louder or slower. The chances are that you don't need this, you may just understand if it's explained in a different way. Once you've cracked it, your ability may be better than someone else who feels they are more able.

I find it really interesting to see people's responses to LDs. In my experience, some people have been more understanding than you could hope for whereas others can go quiet and then perhaps make a sarcastic comment. This is where I feel more should be taught to people about conditions, especially dyspraxia. Often, people, especially children, can end up feeling isolated and/or are bullied because people do not understand why they may find something a challenge or approach it in a different way to others. If more people are aware of the LDs then it could prevent the bullying and not make people feel inferior to others. I think I have only spoken to two or three people who knew what dyspraxia was and this was because they had worked amongst it. This chapter aims to highlight some of the main symptoms of dyspraxia from a down to earth perspective.

In my experiences, often symptoms of LDs overlap. You could take a symptom from dyslexia, such as reversing letters or words: for example reading bed as deb, and someone may also find riding a bike difficult which may come under the umbrella of dyspraxia. It is very difficult to highlight an LD also because personality traits may be just that and could appear as a LD. On the other hand, there may be a LD present and people just think it is a personality trait when it isn't and then this can be a problem. People may see someone as being an attention seeker when they have genuine problems. I have developed a lot of coping strategies over the years and people often tend to do this without realising it. People mask things with humour and I have known people who cannot read, to hide it over many years in embarrassment. I just think some people get to an age where they think they cannot admit to something they feel uncomfortable about. It shouldn't be this way; no one should be ashamed

Where's My Pen?

of a LD. If you are reading this and are a parent who has just discovered your child has a LD, however severe, please don't feel it is a negative thing. Everyone should work together to get to know how to support the person experiencing the LD and increase their knowledge about it.

There are definitely positive aspects of having a LD, a lot of people end up succeeding in whatever they do. It never stopped me doing degrees and going for what I wanted, it just took a bit more patience on my part. The difference is how someone approaches their life and tries not to let challenges defeat them. My advantage of possibly having dyspraxia is that I have so much determination to live life to the full and you really appreciate things that others may take for granted. If you are a parent, the most important thing in my view is to be there with support. Try not to bring out the negative points, try and confirm the positive, encouraging aspects of their personality and bring in humour. This can make life more bearable and the most important medicine as obvious as it sounds, is to laugh about things. There will be times when a person gets frustrated with things they find hard, but other times when they achieve beyond their wildest dreams, like me with this book. There are chapters later in this book which may help people who know someone who suffers with dyspraxia or a LD. I really hope it helps. Remember, there is no rule book, just give it a go and see what happens. The following will hopefully show some of the symptoms of dyspraxia and will help to understand a bit more about the condition.

I could give you all the scientific definitions of dyspraxia, for example, some of them involve the words, impairment, immaturity and organisation of movement (taken from the Dyspraxia Foundation website). However, at first, this could confuse someone who has just been diagnosed with dyspraxia.

If we try and interpret impairment, immaturity, and organisation of movement, it could seem quite daunting with these descriptive words. It may make you feel inferior when you shouldn't at all. This, in basic terms means that you could find it hard to organise how you move, i.e. co-ordinate your body, your thoughts, understanding and instructions.

The actual word 'Dyspraxia' can be split into two words, 'dys' meaning impaired or abnormal, and 'praxis', meaning movement (taken from Wikipedia website). Please don't read the definitions and feel you cannot lead a fulfilling life because you can and there are always ways around challenges you might face in life. It means you may approach not all, but some situations in a slightly different way. The impairment or abnormal movement just means the brain works in a different way, which is not negative and can be positive for lots of reasons (there is a chapter later on which looks at the advantages of being dyspraxic.)

Dyspraxia can be classified in lots of ways and often it can be split into developmental dyspraxia and acquired dyspraxia. Developmental dyspraxia suggests you are born with the condition and

Where's My Pen?

acquired dyspraxia can occur if somebody has experienced a brain injury and/or a stroke for example. This can then cause dyspraxic symptoms.

Hopefully as this book progresses, you may come up with your own interpretation of the condition which is absolutely fine and may make it easier to understand. Some of you will be reading this because, like others you may not know what it is and think that someone you know has it. Others like me may experience it and others may just be interested in it. It took me a while to decide whether to write about personal feelings but then I thought if it does happen to help someone then that suits me down to the ground. My aim of this book is to provide a down to earth perspective and I am not claiming to know everything there is to know about dyspraxia. I am not competing with any authors to be better than anyone; I would just like to add to any help that is out there. The one thing I strongly believe in is that organisations should not try and criticise each other all the time but work together to come up with the most important result-helping people with LDs. Take the politics out and let the genuine help go a long way.

One of the first aspects of dyspraxia is that it is often a hidden condition and you may meet someone and think there is nothing different about them compared to others. It may however be that when faced with learning a new skill like riding a bike, the co-ordination could be really difficult to fathom. Previous descriptions have included the term 'clumsy syndrome' and I would describe myself as clumsy (that's fine with me though!).

If I look back, to when I was in primary school, I was always a scatty child. I would drop things and rush what I was doing. My mum would always say to me, "Sarah concentrate on what you're doing". Like any other child who obviously knows everything (or thinks they do!) I would say, "Stop going on at me!" Quite obviously she was only doing what mums do best, caring for their child. Thinking about it, it sounds a bit corny but I always did feel inferior to everyone else. I felt lucky with what I had and my situation but I always questioned my ability to learn new skills, which looking back now makes complete sense. I was always able to achieve academically but there would be something stopping me reaching my full potential. I remember always saying to people that my brother was very intelligent but I was the one who always had to work hard to achieve something. I got there in the end but it just used to take me a while. This also makes sense now as well. My hand-writing was always a mess in school and when it came to drawing I would struggle to transfer the ideas from my head onto paper. I would want to see my idea on paper as quickly as possible but this would mean rushing it and then ruining it. I remember in art we had to do a piece on the theme of litter. I had this idea of doing packets of crisps with arms and legs and different drawings on a similar theme. I was excited about my idea but when I looked at it on the paper, the idea had not surfaced in the way I wanted it to. My friend would be drawing with

Where's My Pen?

articulation and precision and would finish her piece beautifully. There would be me in a frustration with several scrunched up pieces of paper after just five minutes of art. I remember doing a drawing of a big map, again at school and was really enthusiastic to colour it in and produce something to impress the teacher. It was a nightmare as I spent hours on it only to have to do it all again. Never mind, it was only a drawing in the grand scheme of things.

I was very sporty and always have been. I will never lose the active side to me. I played badminton and ended up playing for Yorkshire schools from about the age of twelve. I loved meeting new people and entering the tournaments although again I realise now there was much more potential there than I actually showed. I would get very tired very quickly and suffer from a lot of headaches during games. I wondered why it was only me that it happened to and not others. I put it down to the fact that I was born with a lazy eye which meant some of the muscles around my eye were weak and this put strain on them when playing badminton. Also, the lights were very bright in the sports halls and so I thought must have been the reason. I think looking back, the reason I reached a plateau with badminton was that I found it hard to keep up with the people who overtook me quickly in terms of faster reaction times and better co-ordination. Perhaps the headaches were as a result of my brain having to work harder to judge the game and respond quickly to the opponent. I can't say I was really bad as I would not have played for my county but I did reach a stage where

I wasn't keeping up with others of my age. This wasn't a problem in the end as my commitment to school exams had to come first to playing badminton.

I remember wanting to play hockey and so I decided to join the hockey team. My difficulties never made me avoid games, it just made me more determined to try them. However, I was put onto the pitch in the second half of a hockey match against one of the top Sheffield schools. When the ball was passed to me I ended up stepping on it as I couldn't keep up with looking for other team members, trying to hit the ball and looking for spaces to pass the ball to. How did people do all this? It was frustrating but I think I was attracted more to the individual sports so I didn't let others down when I found it difficult. I ended up having a go at badminton, athletics, rounders (which I know was a team game as well but I enjoyed it!), gymnastics and a bit of tennis.

Anyway, what's the relevance of me going about all this? Well, from these couple of paragraphs come some of the symptoms of dyspraxia. The first few mentioned highlight a **DIFFICULTY WITH CONCENTRATION**. I mentioned that my mum used to tell me to focus on what I was doing. I would always be on the next part of the task before completing the first bit. This then transferred to activities like cooking. I would sprawl all the ingredients out in a mess and end up having no specific plan. I would get in a muddle with the recipe and then I would get frustrated and upset

Where's My Pen?

because I couldn't do it. Then if someone tried to help me I think I would take my frustration out on them because I didn't understand why I couldn't do something I thought should have been simple. If the brain has a short attention span, then it cannot focus on each stage of an activity so it is harder to complete a task. This is why people can start lots of tasks but not finish them. Of course, this can have repercussions in school because it's not that the ability is not there, it is just that the poor concentration means information is not processed and stored in the brain as effectively.

DIFFICULTY WITH CO-ORDINATION can also be an issue with dyspraxia. This is a big part of the condition and it comes in all shapes and forms. Someone said to me, "I thought dyspraxia was when people fall over and you don't fall over". There are many severities and presentations when thinking about a difficulty with co-ordination. For example, one child could fall over or find going up the stairs so hard to co-ordinate that they have to go on hands and knees. However, someone else may find this okay but struggle with another activity. It can also present in situations where you have to take instructions and put them into practice. For instance, I went to a climbing wall and was really looking forward to having a go. When the instructor showed us how to attach the rope to the carabina, I just could not take the instruction, copy it and then do the same thing. He ended up saying to me: "you're not getting this are you?" and I felt really stupid. It just so happened that my friends picked it up quickly and so I stood out. It took me so much longer than other people to do things. I got there in the end but the frustration is wondering whether people will trust me if I have the problems. The positive aspect of this is that I am aware of my boundaries so I make sure I don't put myself or others in danger.

Another activity I found hard was riding a bike. I was able to ride a bike but when it came to co-ordinating more than one task on a bike then it was tricky. I did my cycling proficiency test and we had to look over our shoulder, then wait for cars, then go and there was a lot to think about. Again, co-ordinating my thoughts mentally while trying to balance physically was not easy. Let's say it was not as easy as riding a bike! Each task on its own was okay but putting it all together was a lot harder.

Swimming was also a struggle. I loved the water but the water didn't love me. One of my memories was that I had to tread water in a school lesson, and I found it especially difficult to carry it out compared with others. The teacher was really horrible and made me cry as a result because I was in the deep end and could not stay above the water. He forced us to tread water for what seemed like forever and it did put me off swimming for a while. I was in the group for extra tuition and felt a bit stupid, as I had no confidence. I was okay at breaststroke but it was front crawl, which was hard. The controlling of arms, legs and breathing were not easy. It isn't easy as a general rule, but I couldn't grasp it all.

Where's My Pen?

Another activity was skiing, well this was very amusing! It wasn't until I was older and an adult that I first tried skiing. I felt like a poor version of Bridget Jones if anyone has seen the film. I had, let's say, a bit of trouble keeping upright on the dry ski slope. I kept falling backwards and I am laughing whilst typing this bit. My friends were going about it like they had been doing it for years and then it was me who happened to fall over going down the slope. Oh well, worse things could have happened, there were no broken bones so that was a relief! Things like that did upset and still do upset me but I just get back on my horse (or is that skis?) again and keep going. I think that's the only way otherwise it defeats you.

DIFFICULTY WITH SPATIAL AWARENESS can also be a challenge. In simple terms this means judging distances and speeds of objects or people within the space around us and being able to react to these in the appropriate way. When I was talking about sport it is interesting that I had strength in an individual sport rather than a team sport. I have always enjoyed working in a team situation, but when it came to spatial awareness, it was tricky. Being aware of spaces to pass in hockey, then being aware of other players and being in control of my own skill was obviously too much for my brain to comprehend. A lot of people whether they are dyspraxic or not may find this difficult but people without dyspraxia may process the information quicker and respond quicker as a result. Spatial awareness then applies to a lot of team sports like netball, football, and basketball.

Additional to spatial awareness, which can affect judgement, is the way we follow balls and objects with our eyes. I mentioned earlier about getting headaches whilst playing badminton. Well, as I got older I realised that my muscles in my eyes were not working together properly. My vision was great with each individual eye but working together was a lot harder. This used to tire my eyes and then I think it lead to the headaches. Looking back now it shows that the brain has to co-ordinate movement of the eyes and so often people with dyspraxia may have muscle problems or **FIND IT HARD TO TRACK OBJECTS** like balls or tracking words on a page when reading. They may find it easy to read the actual words but then get tired easily from reading longer lengths of information. The difficulty with tracking can lead to challenges with throwing and catching.

Another big challenge for someone with dyspraxia is a difficulty with **COMMUNICATION SKILLS**. I always worried that I could never get out what I wanted to say. I always had so much to say but I prepared my words and then when they came out they made no sense. I was told I mumbled and was very quiet, which did a world of good to my self esteem (not!). I would always feel like the outsider in social situations and feel like I was on the outside looking in. I was always better having a few friends who knew me really well and then they couldn't shut me up! I think this is a very important element of dyspraxia, which will be useful for people who do not know what it is. Within dyspraxia you can have verbal dyspraxia, which in simple terms means you can't co-ordinate your brain's intention with what actually comes out of your mouth. There were so many times I would think that I didn't explain things in the way that I meant or wanted to. Then I would worry for ages that I had offended someone and end up thinking no one liked me. My thinking and worrying wasn't useful to me at all but at the time I didn't know the reason for it.

DIFFICULTY WITH HANDWRITING, as mentioned earlier, could be an indicator of dyspraxia although it doesn't mean that everyone who struggles with their handwriting must be dyspraxic. A lot has been mentioned about co-ordination and in this case the brain has to coordinate several movements to write a page of work. I went for an informal chat at a dyslexia centre and they said they didn't think I was dyslexic but thought because I didn't have much control over my pen grip this could indicate dyspraxia. The reason being that joints can be hyper mobile so it is difficult to hold them in one position for a long time without them getting tired. This explains the dent in my finger after writing for long periods of time. (See the chapter on dyspraxia and posture for further explanation of hyper mobility). This may also relate to people finding it hard to stay on the line of a piece of paper if there are no line guides. Again, the control is not there so it goes uphill or downhill.

With poor handwriting also comes **LACK OF ORGANISATION OF WORK.** Again, I always had the intention of being neat and organised but it never turned out that way. I would sit down with a blank piece of paper and think, right this time I am going to organise my file and date everything, put page numbers on for example. The problem came that it took me so long to do this that I couldn't keep up with everything else going on in the class. It would end up a mess as I would try and finish the piece of work. Then it would end up loose in my bag and out of order. This had a knock on effect when it came to revising for exams. I would look at all my notes and they wouldn't really make any sense. I would then end up referring to textbooks as they were neater but would end up reading irrelevant and large amounts of information. This wasted a lot of time and explained why I would work for longer periods and still achieve the same grade.

It was hard during lessons when I had to copy off the board/overhead projector. I had to try and take down all the information so my handwriting would suffer as a result of writing so fast. I then couldn't absorb information the teacher was telling us. An easy solution, which would have really helped me, was if I had been given printouts of the lessons. This way I could have tried to absorb some of the information more easily. When I had to revise for exams it was like starting over again and having to re-learn everything. Throughout university, in theory I could have not attended lectures, as I couldn't retain any of the information they taught us. I know

Where's My Pen?

this is a bit of an exaggeration, but it was hard to remember anything and put it in context of the subject matter we were learning about.

Just to re-cap a few elements of dyspraxia are:

- Difficulty with co-ordination resulting in falling over.

- Difficulty riding a bike, driving and cooking.

- Emotional/Behavioural problems sometimes leading to low self-esteem/depression.

- Difficulty with spatial awareness in sports or activities.

- Difficulty with fine motor skills like writing/drawing/colouring in.

- Difficulty with household tasks and putting things in a sequence.

- Slower information processing when taking/giving instructions.

- Not being able to transfer ideas down on paper when doing an exam for example.

- Difficulty tracking an object like a ball or writing on a page. May have to re-read a page or lines of writing.

- Difficulty with short term memory and retaining information.

This is a brief overview of some of the elements of dyspraxia and the following chapters will hopefully help to clarify some in more detail. I hope there are useful suggestions which may help you decide how to help someone get a diagnosis, support them or just increase your knowledge. This is not meant to be a negative list, it just shows some of the challenges people may face.

Where's My Pen?

Chapter Three: Children and Dyspraxia

The two following chapters focus on children and dyspraxia. Again, I am not claiming to be an expert on the condition, but hope to provide some information which may be useful. Often with books, you may read them and think, okay I know what it is, but is there anything realistic and practical I could try with my child? Well, hopefully the suggestions may help. If they do not look very helpful to you personally, perhaps it will give you an idea to do your own or motivate you to try something new. I have worked with children and adults with dyspraxia so this has helped me understand the condition in other people as well as how I feel about the condition.

Birth to Early Years

From my experiences of talking to parents, dyspraxia can be detected at any age. There can be subtle signs during early years and often birth could involve complications such as babies being premature, having a lack of oxygen, which could result in symptoms of dyspraxia. Very often it may not be picked up in children until they are older. However, parents can look back and think of things their child may have done which would be indicative of dyspraxia. There is a theory that people with LDs may have missed the crawling phase when they were babies and also not lost some of the reflexes they are supposed to lose at certain ages. Babies may bum shuffle at a young age. I could research lots of journal articles and quote lots of authors but I didn't want this book to be like that. I wanted it to be a down to earth perception of dyspraxia. Please consult a professional or read another more detailed book for clarity on this matter about crawling and losing reflexes.

Feeding can be another problem. My mum said when I was younger I went into hospital and the nurses were amazed at the way I was trying to feed myself because I was so messy. I was so determined to do it but I got it everywhere, (I haven't changed!). Feeding can be messy and control of a knife and fork can become troublesome. Dropping of food and missing mouths may occur (although this can be normal with a lot of babies/toddlers).

As a child gets older, it can become apparent that they take longer with learning new skills. I was able to walk but I always clung onto my mum's hand and wouldn't let go as I thought I would fall over. As mentioned earlier, it took me longer to learn to swim and have the confidence. This isn't to say just because someone finds these things difficult they are definitely dyspraxic, but it could be indicative. It may become clear that a child is clumsier than normal and not able to focus on things. Also, they may start lots of activities and not finish them off. It could lead to a mess of lots of activities but nothing completed. Also, it may be that a child is not able to play with a toy and develop ideas surrounding the toy. They may not know how to work it or need

Where's My Pen?

stimulation all the time from another person or source. If they are directed they will find it a lot easier to do things, but left alone it will be hard.

One aspect I have experienced during work is children who experience hand flapping and fidgeting. I remember I used to go for a cuddle with my mum or dad when I was little and I could never lie still. I would feel irritable and a weird ache as though I couldn't stay in one place. Often people get annoyed with fidgeting but I couldn't help it and still can't. I didn't hand flap and not all children with dyspraxia will do this but some may experience it. Children may find it very hard to keep track of their movement and require extra effort to regulate their movements compared to others. It may also be that sensory stimulation is exaggerated in two ways. A child may be over-sensitive to taste and touch. For example, I remember being an awkward child as I couldn't taste fizzy drinks. Perhaps I just plain didn't like them but thinking back, the taste was too strong for me and used to make me feel physically uncomfortable. Birthday parties were tricky as I always ended up being the only one drinking a lot of milk or still drinks. I grew out of it as my taste buds developed but children can often appear fussy in eating and drinking. They may also hypo-sensitive to foods, so not taste flavours as much as others. This could cause them to be fussy about certain foods and tastes.

Difficulties with skills such as cutting and colouring in could stand out as a problem. I was left-handed so I found cutting a nightmare anyway. I had left handed scissors but they were very blunt so I would never be very neat. All these aspects just culminate in frustration and having to take longer to do things. Using a knife and fork would be hard as it was difficult to cut things. Lack of strength in my fingers and hands meant I would try and tear my food instead of cutting it. It never stopped me from eating the food let me tell you, but it was a bit messy. One important aspect of these techniques is to remember that it may not be lack of strength children have in their fingers whilst using a knife and fork for example, it is the motor planning of the movement. This means the brain engaging in the movement of holding the fork, cutting the food and lifting it to the mouth.

It could also be that, coincidentally, the child does have weakness as well, but a lot of the time it may be the motor planning which is the main problem. This is why thicker grips for knives and forks may come in handy. It requires less control over the knife and fork, requiring less planning of the movement. Whilst eating, it may come apparent that children are tearing their meat if they eat it. This again, is because it requires more planning to place the knife in a certain position to then cut continuously to break a piece of meat up. It is a lot easier and quicker for the brain to tear it and quickly eat it. This can obviously vary amongst individuals but it may be useful to monitor how your child eats and if there are ways to help them find it easier. Hopefully this may help you understand if you have a child who is not eating certain types of food or loves another type of food which is soft on

Where's My Pen?

the palate. Certain textures of food may be easier to eat for some children so just try your best to support this. It may not stand out too much as a lot of children tend to be fussy about their eating anyway. Grips for knives and forks which are colourful and trendy may make children feel more comfortable using them.

In terms of co-ordination as a child gets older, dressing for school involving top buttons on blouses/shirts and doing up laces can be a problem. These are techniques often taken for granted that children will be able to do. However, it can be really tricky for a child to get their head around doing laces. We do tend to be blessed with a lot of Velcro nowadays but it would be good if children could try and learn. Try and split it into small sections when teaching them. Instead of saying, "you should be able to do your laces", have a go at setting them small targets. For example, 1) do the first part of laces like getting shoes on and then 2) putting the laces over one another. If anyone is faced with a complete challenge it can often be overwhelming. If it is broken down into small sections it is easier. When writing this book, if someone said, right you've got to finish it in two days it would make me worried. However, I give myself small tasks to do and find that I do more than the task I set. It's not putting too much pressure on the brain to achieve too much. If the brain is bombarded with too much information at once, it can cause panic and then nothing gets done as the brain then switches off. I know I have gone off on a tangent but I think this can be applied to lots of situations with children and dyspraxia. If you say to a child, get up, get dressed, clean your teeth and then have breakfast this can be very overwhelming. A child may remember the last instruction and forget the others which may make them look like they are just standing there when really they are trying to process information about all the tasks given. If you say get out of bed first, let them do that, then tell them to get dressed etc. then it is split up into small tasks. I know this sounds obvious, but it can then be applied to more complex tasks like academic tasks in school. I'm sure a child could describe exactly how to do a task, but it may become a lot harder in practice.

In terms of motor planning, for children they may struggle in physical education (PE), especially with team games. Some children may be naturally skilled at football. However, there are a lot of aspects of the game which could be tricky for someone with dyspraxia. Looking for other players may be hard as it can be difficult for children to judge distances and spaces. If someone has to think quickly then process information about where to pass the ball, it might be hard to fathom. There are quite a few parts, just like my example of hockey mentioned in this book, to think of when playing the game. It may be that children try and opt out of these games. If a child is self conscious about appearing clumsy or not passing a ball in football then this could lead to bullying. If children experience this then it may affect the way they view sport and as a result see it as a negative experience and avoid it. On the other hand,

Where's My Pen?

sometimes children may practice more because they want to improve and they may become just as good as any other players. Because they find it hard but have the intelligence, their determination may mean their hard work pays off. Often they may become better than some of the children who have ability but don't put it to use.

Children may find it hard to perform certain moves in PE where co-ordination comes into play. It may be an idea to practice throwing and catching with a bigger ball to get used to the actual process of it, then gradually reducing the size of the ball with time. If you introduce different sizes and shapes at the beginning of learning, then it could be confusing. Running could also be challenging in terms of co-ordinating arms with legs. It could be that children find themselves tripping up, I know I used to stand on the back of peoples' ankles by accident-bet I was popular!

When children are older, the signs of dyspraxia may not be as obvious because they may find coping strategies or cover things up to avoid embarrassment, which is why I think it can often be a hidden condition. I was so shy that I would never have admitted to struggling at things at school. I just worked hard to try and achieve my work. I was above average at spelling and certain aspects of my work were okay so alarm bells didn't ring immediately. The main aspect for me was the organisation of my work. That was hard and I was not the neatest person. I would get frustrated that I couldn't write like everyone else. When it came to reading I was good at it but could never remember what I had read. I would become distracted, lose my place and have to re-read a chapter. Children with dyspraxia can have different problems and may vary with their abilities. I have come across children who have an overlap of dyslexia and dyspraxia so reading of words and spelling can be hard for them to fathom. Other people like myself, can read really quickly but it is retaining and re-telling the story which is tough to do. If a child is embarrassed about finding something hard, they can quite easily pretend they have finished reading something in their head and when questioned as a class, just not answer. This can often be overlooked.

It is a case that children can learn in different ways. If instructions are not clear in their intention it may be really hard for children to understand what they have to do. Again, it could appear that a child is not doing their work, but they are trying to process in their mind what they need to be doing. They may then ask their friends and possibly copy off someone else. This is where I think it is really important for teachers to be aware of these learning differences. Understandably it is really hard to be aware of every child in a class of thirty but if they understood about dyspraxia, they could make a few adjustments which could have a big effect. All I really needed was some extra prompts whether it was verbal or quick demonstrations. Explanation in a different way would and still does make a difference to taking information in. Once children understand what they have to do then often they

Where's My Pen?

will be able to finish a task very well and often quicker than others. Hopefully the tips in the next chapter are useful in terms of reading and writing.

Low self esteem can often be present in a person with a LD, often leading to a self deprecating nature. This means that a child may put themselves down because if they find some things hard, they could assume everything will be the same. Behaviour may present in different forms. One child may act the comedian as this deters away from their learning and they forget about their schoolwork. Another form of behaviour may be shyness and withdrawing from situations. Again, if they find a situation hard and have less confidence, they may assume this will often be the case. Therefore, you could understand why a child may protect themselves from any embarrassment or peer pressure. I was like this to a certain extent. It would upset me and frustrate me if I found something hard, like swimming. I would be determined to get better but I did find it really hard and it made me very anxious. I had to battle with myself not to miss and avoid doing the task which was a challenge to me. Other children may become aggressive or attention seeking in different forms to pent their frustration. It could be a way of trying to release the frustration of feeling different from others or left out. I don't want this to make it sound like this is what all children with dyspraxia feel like. Personalities will handle situations in different ways so you may have a child who does not present in any of these ways. It is like any process, humans react to things very differently so there may be certain situations which are easier than others. It can be the same for a LD. People will handle situations in different ways but it is just important to find the right support for that child at the time. If this isn't in place, there could be repercussions later in life when the frustration builds and may come out in different forms of behaviour.

Behaviour can sometimes be affected when someone suffers from dyspraxia and tantrums can surface. This is a tricky one because does this make every child dyspraxic as potentially, all children could have tantrums? No, it will normally go along with other signs, which may seem a bit different for a child of a certain age. When I was younger I went through a period of having tantrums and looking back I wasn't sure why and my parents don't know why either. I remember cutting a big hole in the towel in the bathroom and then pretending it wasn't me! Looking back, I have no idea what was going on. However, it could have been due to the frustration or not having attention. It sounds like it was an attention-seeking act although I can't remember feeling like I wanted the attention. The point of this section is for parents or friends to remember there is usually an explanation to the behaviour. It is not always easy to find it out if the child finds it hard to express themselves. Maybe ask teachers or friend's parents if they have mentioned anything. They may open up to other people. Try to be patient with them-it isn't always their fault. It is a really hard thing, (I am not a parent so I am not in a position to give out advice in parenting but from my experience I might have told

Where's My Pen?

a friend about my problems.) Sometimes children can be really open with their family but this can vary. Remember that it may be hard for the child to express verbally or when writing something down. Therefore, frustration can manifest in several forms-shyness, withdrawal, anger, frustration for example. Try and empathise and think of a situation, which you find frustrating but cannot change. I find it hard that I can never change the fact my brain is the way it is but I can adopt different coping strategies and positive approaches to things. Try and make situations easier for the child whilst at the same time giving them independence (hard balance I know).

Once children become teenagers I think they can be even more aware of themselves and the pressure put on them by others. This is the time when a LD can be a sensitive subject. Some teenagers may openly talk about it where others may feel embarrassed and not want to stand out. It is a very personal thing to the individual and this may change over time as they get older. For me if someone had clarified where my problems were coming from I think I would have been relieved. Again, the main thing to think about is trying to step back and support them in the way you think is best. There is no rule book but just try and be patient. Hopefully the following chapter will help give some ideas to help.

Chapter Four: Hints and Tips For Children And Teenagers

In this chapter there may be parts which you will use, others may not work for you. Don't worry, there are no specific rules, just give some a go and see what happens! If you do not understand things written in this chapter then ask someone to help you, it is nothing to be ashamed of if you ask for help, just a sign of maturity and intelligence!

- The first part is about reading. The important thing to remember is not to put too much pressure on yourself as reading is tiring for anyone so take regular breaks as you will take in more information. It can be frustrating to have to re-read something over and over until it sticks in your brain. Use one of the bookmarks to write down a brief summary of what has happened in the story so far in-case you have forgotten or you have a longer break from the story.

- Find books with larger print, understandably children or you may be embarrassed if they feel peer pressure but they/you could always just read these books at home if it is a problem. It is nothing to be embarrassed about but people feel differently and react in different ways.

- See if you can tell people little bits about the story so your brain is working to remember things.

Where's My Pen?

- Try not to avoid reading as I used to do. It was so tiring for me but if you keep reading in small chunks then this is good practice. The brain needs exercise to work more effectively like your muscles need work to make them stronger.

- Have regular breaks instead of feeling pressure to read a lot. However, there may be times when you want to read for longer, so just enjoy it!

- If you are reading a book at school and it is also a film, try and watch it. Even though films are slightly different to books, you can still get the idea of the story from it. This helps with the understanding of them.

- Do not put pressure on yourself; people with dyspraxia are usually of average or above average intelligence. Try and just think that your brain just works in a different way and that can be a positive thing!

- Depending on what stage of reading, perhaps use your finger as a guide or a ruler. This is not something you want to rely on but it may help for a while.

- If your eyes hurt, tell a parent or carer and you may need your eyes testing. Glasses or contact lenses may help to improve reading and tracking/looking at objects.

Writing

- There a lots of pen grips you could use to help with writing. You can get some fun colours! This may help your hand hurt less if it gets sore from writing a lot. Try practising the technique of using a pen in sand as this will help strengthen your pen grip/paintbrush grip and improve co-ordination hopefully.

- Again, like reading, write in small chunks. Don't worry about the whole piece of writing. I used to want to finish the whole thing quickly so I could see what it was going to be like. Just concentrate on each bit at time. Try and write down a plan of ideas at the beginning although get someone to help if this is hard to do. It may make your mind feel like it is thinking in a better order. You could record ideas on a video or tape etc. if you cannot put them onto paper easily. A lot of people with dyspraxia find they have the ideas in their head but find it hard to write them on paper. Don't worry if this happens, you could tell someone the ideas and they could help and write them down for you.

- Try not to get too frustrated if you cannot write ideas down. Everyone finds that some days they can write a lot and others they cannot write anything. From talking with my mum, she said I used to find it hard to write down bullet points about the main issues of something I had read about. If this is the case for you, please ask

Where's My Pen?

someone to help. Just try and enjoy it, easier said than done I know-but there are several people who suffer with dyspraxia who have written books. Don't give up! Keep going, it will be worth the hard work!

- Do not be afraid to ask for help. Someone I spoke to, suggested a sign of an intelligent person, is someone who asks questions or asks for help-do not worry! We cannot know everything and people know different things. This is a good thing because we can all teach each other.

- If you find you are not writing enough, then each time you do a piece of work try and write a little bit more. Again, take it one step at a time otherwise it may make you worried about it.

- Use rhymes to help you remember things in your work. The sillier the rhymes are the better may retain them. For example, people remember the alphabet more when they sing it- this helps the brain to store the information about the alphabet better than if you had to write it down.

Tidying Up and Keeping Organised

- Find someone who can help you make boxes which are colourful and you can stick pictures on. These boxes may help you keep tidy and put all your things in.

- Try and put labels on them like shoes, jewellery, football things for example.

- Have a little box for any keys you may have and put it by the door where it is safe and secure. Make sure you keep putting the keys in there so you will always know where they are-one less thing to worry about.

- If you keep losing your pens, try and have colourful grips so you can recognise them and find them more easily.

- If you find using a diary difficult or boring, you could decorate a notebook and write what you do day by day. Try and concentrate on one day at a time so things do not get stressful.

- Try and get things ready for school the night before. This means you can have a few extra minutes in bed! You will feel less worried in the morning if everything is ready the night before.

- Every now and again get someone to help you or do it on your own, but sort out your room and

Where's My Pen?

make sure your belongings are in the boxes you made. If they have got mixed up don't worry about it. Just try and put it right with help or on your own.

- See if you can get a bag with different compartments in so you can put certain things in certain places. I have had a bag with one big pocket in and I can never find things when I need them. It takes me ages to find my pens and things. You could have a separate bag for PE for example so you always know where your kit is.

- Try and put music on while you tidy up and make it fun. Invite a friend to help you sort things and sing/dance while you do it. Make sure you do not get distracted, but you could combine both and have fun!

- Set yourself a reward at the end of the task whether it is watching your favourite programme on television or eating something you enjoy. This will keep you tidying up and finishing the task.

- When you are thinking of what you need for school try and break it down into little bits. For example, if you are going swimming try and think of the whole process. I go into the changing rooms so I need my swimming things, then I may want to swim underwater so I need my goggles-and so on. This may make things clearer in your mind. It may help or it may not- just give it a go!

- Have a go at the activities on the following pages. They might really help you organise yourself. If you are a teenager and feel you are too old for them, then design your own as I'm sure you will have the intelligence to!

- Photocopy the page or draw your own star (you could also trace it with help).

- For every day, write what you need for school.

- Then colour and design it like you want to. There are no rules, just what helps you!

- Put it on the wall so it reminds you to remember everything for school!

Where's My Pen?

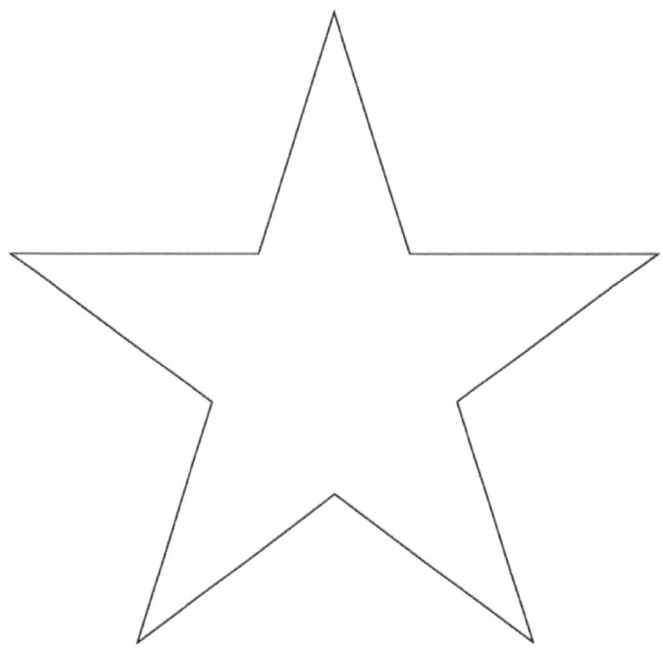

Bookmark which can be photocopied or traced:

- Get someone to help you laminate the bookmark.

- Get a non permanent marker and write about each chapter when reading a book.

- Or……stick a post it note on the bookmark and write a summary of the chapter, whatever works better for you!

- Wipe the information off the bookmark when going onto the next chapter.

- If you find it hard to understand the instructions just ask for help!

- Make it as colourful as you want it to be.

Where's My Pen?

Photocopy or write out your own page to help others understand about you. You don't have to do this if you feel uncomfortable; you could make your own details up!

WHAT DYSPRAXIA MEANS TO ME:

WHAT HELP YOU COULD GIVE ME:

WHAT I AM GOOD AT:

SOMETHING I WOULD LIKE TO TRY IN MY LIFE:

These are just ideas, you can design your own and put colour on it to make it a bit cooler!

A guide for what is dyspraxia?

DYSPRAXIA IS................

- Difficulty processing thoughts and actions.

- Difficulty with co-ordination, both mentally and physically. e.g. riding a bike/tying laces/using knife and fork/handwriting/fine motor skills.

- Difficulties transferring thoughts/ideas to paper.

- Difficulties taking more than one instruction at once.

- Finding it hard to organise things.

- Difficulty with communication and speech at times.

- Falling over, tripping over objects/low tone-posture.

- Low self esteem as a result of the above.

Where's My Pen?

None of the suggestions in this chapter are rocket science, they are just common sense but it is sometimes hard to think of them. You may find your own way of coping with things and this is great so the important thing is not to give up! Good luck with everything whether you are a parent/carer or child with dyspraxia. I really hope you have found something in this chapter useful or you can now explain it a bit more to someone else.

Chapter Five: Being an Adult with Dyspraxia

As an adult, I have been quite amazed at the complete mixture of responses when talking about LDs whether it is dyslexia, dyspraxia, or autism for example. Some people seem genuinely interested and then others seem to want to challenge you and try and make you feel like you're making things up. I am not seeking attention by talking about dyspraxia. Obviously I would love attention from this book but the attention I want is from people reading it and getting some benefit from it. I sometimes think that it can be harder for adults to cope if they suffer with a LD. This is not because they cannot get through life without achieving, quite the contrary; it is the way some people perceive or do not know enough about different conditions. Even people who know me well, at times, cannot see what could be dyspraxia and what could not be. I have a personal feeling that this is such a shame that lots of intelligent people do not know what some LDs are. This is not their fault in terms of they haven't had the need to know about them or come across someone who experiences dyspraxia. However, if they did learn more when they were younger, it wouldn't just be luck of knowing about a condition, it would be more of an accepted thing.

As an adult and having gone through experiences as a child and adult with possible dyspraxia, I decided to write to Gordon Brown to say that I felt schools need more awareness on dyspraxia for both teachers and pupils. The reason I did this was

Where's My Pen?

really to put my point across. I'm quite aware that I wouldn't have a massive impact on the world, but I just wanted to air my views. I did receive a letter back and it said more information was being taught to teachers in order to increase their understanding of LDs. I really hope this is true and they didn't just say it for effect. Hopefully in ten years time, LDs will be an accepted part of everyday life and awareness will be greater; fingers crossed.

This chapter will cover different aspects of the adult with dyspraxia. I think there are probably quite a few people who may be dyspraxic but go undiagnosed. I can think of a few people I know who may be dyspraxic, without tarring everyone with the same brush. It is a tricky one as often dyspraxic symptoms could also seem like traits that all people possess. For example, losing possessions can happen with lots of people. However, it is when there are quite a few other dyspraxic symptoms which have an impact on someone's life. Another interesting point to note is that often adults have already developed coping strategies so it is not as evident. I hide a lot of my difficulties not because I embarrassed, I have just developed ways around different challenges. For example, if I do not organise myself then I will be a nightmare. Therefore, I make sure aspects of my life are organised. To another person they may just see that I am organised. They will not see all the effort I have put in beforehand. I make sure I am aware of organising myself, which is often really hard and can be stressful at times.

As you have already read, I did struggle as a child but the dyspraxia wasn't picked up. It was only about a year ago that I found out that there could be a possibility of dyspraxia. There may be people reading this who are in a similar situation and may think, "oh well, I've coped this far, there's no point getting help". It is obviously your choice, but since I have known what it could be, it has really helped and I have found different therapies which have helped me cope. It is never too late to seek help and I can assure you that someone may give you at least one idea which could help with aspects of your life without compromising your independence. It seems at teenage years that as a child matures, things can get a bit easier, but then pressures of living independently become quite tricky. The following aspects of life can become tricky:

Household chores
Organising aspects of work/studying
Emotional issues/relationships
Driving
Socialising/integrating in a conversation

Again, writing about my experiences just hopefully demonstrates a real life experience whilst struggling. I did my A-levels at a sixth form college and there wasn't as much teaching structure. I found it hard and tiring to organise all the work for the subjects. To cut a long story short I came out with lower grades than I worked for. Admittedly alcohol and boys began to become more and more a part of my life but I felt I had still put in a lot of hours but didn't get the grades to reflect this.

Where's My Pen?

Looking back, I think a sixth form school would have given me more structure perhaps. This is not to say the college wasn't good because it was, but for learning styles I found it quite tough. I got over the disappointment of my A-level results and was able to do a sport degree.

Little did I know at the time that perhaps a sports degree would be one of the most challenging courses in terms of co-ordination. However, I have and do love sport so that was why I applied. There were some aspects of the course like swimming for example that were more challenging than others.

When it came to swimming, this was to be entertaining. Everyone else could dive apart from me and every week I dreaded it. Once again I stood out, "and the award for champion belly flopper of the year goes to.....Sarah!" Great, I just loved the look of frustration as the county swimmers finished their 300 lengths in 30 seconds and there's me struggling to do 8 lengths let alone 300. It was quite amusing looking back though.

Our teacher was quite strict let's say and she put me in the lane with all the county swimmers, I think so she could have a giggle for the afternoon. Funnily enough I ended up getting 40% for that module, the pass mark and the lowest in the class. As mentioned earlier, it was the co-ordination I found hard. I could do breast stroke but never front crawl. This was tricky to try and breathe at the same time as co-ordinating arms and legs. Oh well, it was okay, as dance was next. Great, I have to say I loved dancing in theory but in practice it was quite different than throwing some shapes on the dance floor on a night out. If I was dancing in my own way it would be in time as I was always very musical. However, we come onto another symptom of dyspraxia; that is taking in instructions. Admittedly taking lots of instructions during dance is hard for anyone but when your mind has to repeat those instructions about ten thousand times it does get a bit tricky. Mental block springs to mind and again you can see how it all makes sense but putting it into practice, well that is another thing.

I really enjoyed all the sports but wasn't that great at them. I was fine at badminton as I had played for so many years, but issues with spatial awareness and co-ordinating certain aspects of sport did make it harder. I just always felt there was a block there- as though I could have done better. Volleyball was a prime example. I loved it but couldn't quite master a few moves. I was fine with the serving as this was quite similar to an over arm badminton serve. However, when it came to keeping the ball in the air, my aim was let's say a bit skew whiff! It was fun though and I suppose that was the main thing.

I managed to finish the degree and achieved a 2.1 with determination. My parents supported me but I had to work very hard for it. I think that is one advantage in a weird kind of way that if you have dyspraxia and you have to work harder at least you feel you have achieved something when you do finally get there. I guess it would be boring if I was a

Where's My Pen?

complete genius and always got everything right in a few minutes!

When I graduated into the real world, this was to be an interesting, let's say learning curve, whichever way you may see it! I was toying between doing physiotherapy or a completely new career. Like a lot of young people searching for a decent career, I found it tough. One day I decided being a recruitment consultant would be good, the next I was going to be a nurse. The day after I would decide to be a sports psychologist and then the days go on… well, I decided to give the recruitment consultant job a go and began on the salary of £9,000. This was not a lot to live on but it was better than nothing. I began a probationary period like a lot of people do and worked within a small office. Not knowing about the dyspraxia at the time it was to be a nightmare and the self esteem began to go in a downward spiral. It began by having to use the phone and I wondered why I couldn't answer the phone and enter data into the computer at the same time. How hard can it be? I was very timid so the phone was not my great friend anyway, and I was surrounded by people who were not very understanding of people making mistakes or being shy. It was an industry where confidence had to shine through or at least appear to anyway! I was wondering why I couldn't even laminate a piece of paper or do something straight forward which then lead to the inferior feeling. When I look back it also makes sense as to why I couldn't process information when talking on the phone and answering queries. I also couldn't think of anything to say in conversations-again, which makes sense as there was a mis-communication with certain parts of my brain! In the end I felt so down that I had to end the job and was just honest to my manager who was actually quite shocked at how much I talked when describing why I found things difficult. It just wasn't the right job for me at all but hey ho, these things happen for a reason I'm sure. The next job I went to involved working for a rugby team. I was a general assistant and so had to organise my workload. My desk looked as though it had a constant tree on it, i.e. a huge pile of paper, which needed sorting out. I always knew what I wanted to do but couldn't quite do it. I was always running around like a stressed person but wasn't actually getting that much work done. I just managed to waste a lot of time and not use my time efficiently. I suppose I perfected the art of making tea as that was something I could do.

One goal that I was determined to conquer was my fear of the phone so I decided to always answer the phone when I could. I did this and it really did improve my confidence. I was still shy but it became more bearable. The ironic thing was that I would always get high phone bills when talking to friends but in a work situation it was tough. Again, I have probably harped on about this but the sheer fact that I found things hard made me face my fear and try my hardest to achieve it. This made me a bit crazy like facing my fear of heights by jumping out of a plane, but I was determined to do it. It's a good feeling when you have tried hard and you get something out of it.

Where's My Pen?

After a while of travelling and having a break, I decided to really go for the physiotherapy attempt at a career. I had always loved working with people and although shy, I did love looking after people and my caring side came out making me more outgoing in certain situations. My determination pulled me through again and before I knew it I was starting a second degree. I did find it hard to organise my work and to cut a long first year short I ended up re-taking an exam in the first year. Practically I had to take in a lot of instructions in theory lectures and practical lectures. This was admittedly meant to be hard but I did struggle overall. I found in lectures I couldn't copy off the board and take in the information. As mentioned earlier, I could have not bothered with the lecture as I had to start again in terms of learning when I came to revise. The lecturer could have explained anything but my mind would start to wander and go away into fairy land. Concentration went, not from want of trying, but it was just tricky. Again, it was determination and I suppose stubbornness not to let it defeat me.

I worked all summer to revise for my re-take and I passed it in the end and went onto my second year. I found with the assignments I was doing, again I struggled with structuring the essays. I wanted to put all the information down and it would never come out right. There was no logical and succinct scientific way of writing for me; it was just a lot of waffle. I knew what I wanted to put down and the ideas connected to the physiotherapy made sense but transferring them across as mentioned earlier was a different kettle of fish. I particularly found one placement hard when I began going into the hospitals. This involved working with children and I really had a desire to work in this area of physiotherapy. I was working in intensive care which was difficult for anyone but I just couldn't cope with all the information and applying it to the situation. Then stress set in and I found it hard to remember my own name let alone anything else. I remember trying to get a wheelchair through a door and one of the physiotherapists saying "god I wouldn't like to see you driving". That did hurt me but it just confirmed to me at the time that I must have been stupid. I was really upset throughout the whole of that placement and my friends must have been very patient with me. Self esteem was at an all time low because I had so much to give potentially but couldn't quite put it into an order or structure. I was told I was too slow at writing notes and the harder I tried the worse it got. Then once again stress reared its ugly head.

Determination took me through to the end of my course and I had two very good placements after my challenging one. I achieved a 2.1 which I was so pleased about and the blessing was that for some reason I could verbally explain things in job interviews. I actually surprised myself and had plenty to talk about. I landed a job in a small hospital in Wales and this was to be the moment when the dyspraxia totally reared its ugly head.

I was concerned about letting lots of my feelings out in this book but if anyone associates with what I

Where's My Pen?

am about to describe please please seek help. There is a way around it and it won't be like that forever. Here goes…. I began my three-month rotations as a junior physiotherapist and was petrified for most of it. It is undoubtedly a learning curve for anyone newly qualifying as a physiotherapist but I somehow felt very different to everyone else. I felt anxious about stupid things and I ended up dreading going into work as I just felt like a fraud. Because my short term memory was bad, I was forgetting my anatomy that I had learnt in first year and I couldn't retrieve the information from my brain that I needed at the time.

It was in my head, I just couldn't communicate it very easily. I did have the strength of working from a holistic approach and I think this is what kept me going as a physiotherapist. When I started the beginning of a breakdown, the other physiotherapists were not concerned by my work and wondered why I was so upset about it all. It all started one morning when I had got so stressed I just couldn't go into work. This will probably sound extremely bizarre, but I couldn't work out something that to a lot of people, was straight forward. Every time I tried to work it out in what I thought was a logical way, I would hit a mental block. Then the spiral of anxiety came, then the "why am I so stupid", thoughts came. After that, the determination would set in and I would seek to find the answer. My friends would try and explain things to me and I still wouldn't get it and just had to accept that my brain worked in a different way. I think this is what has brought on the inferior feeling over the years. It is not so much that I couldn't achieve things eventually; it was why I felt so different to other people. Why did other people make things look so easy? I always found I could do the harder tasks rather than the more straightforward things. Very bizarre! Although, again, now I know what it could be, I just laugh about it and accept it-it's a kind of uniqueness I guess!

Anyway, back to the story of work and the stress/depression. Well, I believe, looking back on everything, my body and mind had taken on so much anxiety and stress from trying so hard to work normally that it had reached shut down phase. The body has a clever way of just giving up on things at certain times. I reached a stage where I believed I couldn't do anything. I couldn't organise cooking, cleaning, work, my driving was hard work. Why was it that every time I achieved something, waiting for me next time would be another failure? I don't mean to feel sorry for myself, I just mean it never worked that I did something and achieved it, did something and achieved. I would work hard and eventually get it, and then I would find something impossible again and so on. It just wasn't adding up and my mindset totally changed. The panic attacks started and all of a sudden I couldn't cope with anything. Now the alien feeling of depression set in and for the first time in my life I didn't want to live. The reason I didn't want to live was because if I couldn't do anything for myself what was the point? Things got so bad that I did genuinely want to get rid of the bad feelings but my family and friends

Where's My Pen?

pulled me through. This I really owe to them as I was not easy to put up with or live with. I had suddenly achieved a physiotherapy degree, but then couldn't do the job I had always wanted to do. What now? All that work and I realised it was all too overwhelming. Everything suddenly became impossible. I never really understood depression before and I think a lot of people perceive it in the wrong way. A doctor told me just to put on a film that made me laugh and I would be fine. This really patronised me as if it was that simple, I would not have ended up in hospital for depression. It has made me realise that it is a complete change of state of mind. Now I am back to my rational, dyspraxic self (is that possible?) I look back and realise that at the time I was convinced that everything I was saying was the truth. I thought nobody liked me and why would anyone want to be my friend if I was so rubbish at everything. I was mid twenties and lots of people treated me as younger. I was so shy at work that I wouldn't say boo to a goose.

When I was off work for depression someone said, "don't worry you were so quiet we hardly knew the difference anyway". Now you can't shut me up! For any shy person reading this, it is one of the worst things you can hear. "You're so quiet aren't you?" If people were not shy then they wouldn't be quiet but everyone is made differently and not everyone can suddenly talk all the time and be loud. I look back now and realise why I held quite a lot of jealousy, not in a mean way, but in a silent, I wish I was good at that way. That's not to say I didn't try a lot of things and attempted them to a degree, I couldn't reach my full potential. A big part also makes sense as to why I never knew what to say because my thoughts wouldn't process quickly enough. I was the quiet one in the background who would say a joke then two seconds later the louder person would say the exact same thing and people would laugh. It was always a battle to feel part of a group and I think that's also why I had few good friends rather than a big group.

The feeling I would describe was like I was on the outside looking in. I was never immersed in anything for fear that I would not understand it or be able to do it. If I had my own time to try something at my own pace then it was a different story. However, under pressure was the worst thing that could happen. It made co-ordination even harder.

If anyone is suffering now as they read this, please seek help. I felt there was never going to be a time when I would feel better. I couldn't get out of bed and it took me so long to have a shower. Now I am very active and writing a book so things cannot be any more different. Hopefully there may be a few handy hints in the next chapter to help you cope with life.

Where's My Pen?

Chapter Six: Tips For Adults Who Have Dyspraxia

This chapter will hopefully help even if only a few pieces of advice are taken in. It aims not to patronise, but to guide you in the right direction if some aspects of life are hard to fathom. Some advice you may read and think you have tried it and it didn't work. Don't worry, pick another piece and try that! It's all trial and error.

Tips to coping with dyspraxia:

- When you have a pang of frustration, take a deep breath and try and laugh about it! (easier said than done I know).

- Lists,lists,lists! It really does work. You might not do all on the list-but you might achieve one. Lists can apply to all situations. Have a go at cooking, but write a list out before and take it in small chunks. Put music on and be conscious of not getting stressed. You will enjoy it more and you will put less pressure on yourself.

- Take life in small chunks. Don't think of the bigger picture as it is too overwhelming. For example, if you find household chores difficult, do small sections of a room, one step at a time. Take cleaning the bathroom as an example. Focus on the bath first and forget the rest. Then do the sink followed by the floor. I know this sounds really obvious but I used to start doing the bath, not finish it, then go onto the sink and get distracted and there ended up being no order. I would then forget what I had and hadn't finished. Just give it a go!

- Talk to people about how you feel-it is not against the law. You'll be surprised at how many people will be willing to help.

- Just by the sheer nature of having dyspraxia you will empathise with other people who find things difficult.

- Why not do at least one thing a day for someone else, one thing a day you enjoy and one thing that you are supposed to do but have been putting off.

- Don't be afraid of asking for help.

- Don't put too much pressure on yourself (anyone who knows me will be saying pot, kettle and black, I know!).

- Try and take advantage of your creative side.

- Everyone has something to offer, fact!

- Try and educate people about dyspraxia, it doesn't have to be over the top.

Where's My Pen?

- Get items which help like pen grips, kettle grippers, for example.

- Never give up because you feel you can't do it. You can it just may take you longer.

- Remember if you find something hard but achieve it in the end it means more than just finding something really easy to do.

- Try and write a book, I have-if it helps someone, great!

- Put dyspraxia into google and see what it comes up with.

- Take your time with things. When you feel stressed, stop, take a deep breath and then carry on!

- Get a stress ball and squeeze it when things are tough.

- Just remember you are allowed days when you are fed up of having the condition but don't let it last more than a day at a time.

- Have a blitz of your room. Keep things in boxes. My mum is great with organisational skills so ask people in the know.
- Put on your favourite song and sing your lungs out. Good stress relief! Don't worry if you get all the words wrong and you're out of tune.

- Remember, corny but true-there is no rule book to life, just suck it and see! (bet you can't put a fruit pastille in your mouth without chewing it!)

- Give someone else who has dyspraxia a piece of advice as everyone has different strengths and weaknesses within dyspraxia.

- Don't worry about the people who say "oh I can't believe people are given all these labels nowadays". Tough, it can be helpful sometimes to know why you find things difficult. Get them to tell you one thing they have a strong opinion on. Then get them to imagine someone really doubting it and being horrible about it. See what they say.

Where's My Pen?

DYSPRAXIA JUST FOR FUN!

Driving – could be interesting!

Yep it's what I've got-please be patient

Sense of humour essential

Pride-don't let it get in the way

Routine-use it sometimes, other times try not to use it and be spontaneous!

Aaaaargh! Things can be a challenge but I will overcome this!

X –Xylophone, what else is there beginning with x (ok, Xanadu etc).

Interesting with initiative – dyspraxic people think outside the box!

Animals and children can be our strong point.

- This is only advice, but why not do something for charity-it does help put things into perspective.

- Don't forget that even if you make a mistake sometimes it turns out better. I once ordered a curry from the wrong place but it ended up being nicer than the one we usually went to. It's like the Worcester sauce advert where she's cooking and thinks that the Worcester sauce is red wine. It actually turns out that everyone loves it more than the wine. So, remember it doesn't always end up bad!

- Write down or type your thoughts out. Sometimes this may help you.

- Tips on writing: Use pen grips – You can try several grips to see which one suits your writing style, have a look on the internet for the Dyspraxia Foundation who could help you. Perhaps buy three or four like me so if I lose them I know I have a spare grip. It was a running joke in my previous job as to who found my missing pen and where I had left it, hence the name of the book! You can get left handed grips as well. Alternatively, get a thicker pen if you do not want a pen grip. I feel you are never too old for something which ultimately helps you to do something more efficient and neater.

- Try and write in small chunks. From my experience I write loads and then just have to start again. Use mind maps/spider diagrams. Put all your thoughts down. Then take each thought and break it down further. Don't look at the whole picture as it will be too overwhelming. This way you can organise your thoughts better. I've been writing this book by jumping all over the place with the order. I have, in the last few days written the chapter headings and I will fit all the relevant information in. If I had done this

Where's My Pen?

at the start it may have saved me time. It isn't a problem, but may be a tip to help you.

- Don't be afraid to ask for advice on structuring your essays or stories. I used to get pulled up on the way I structured things so the lecturer would not be able to read it in a flow. I once did an essay, which was meant to be straightforward but because I found it hard to transfer my thoughts and ideas I got a D for it when I should have got a higher mark. It hurts when you spend the longest time on an essay then you get the lowest mark out of your friends. However, at the same time I try not to dwell on it as we have other things to offer.

- Don't put too much pressure on yourself. People can be so guilty of this.

- Take regular breaks so you come back to it afresh. Do something entirely different in your five minute break. It seems silly to spend that time stressing about the work when you can change thought and come back to it again.

- With reading, concentrate in small chunks so you can absorb the information better. Use a finger as a guide if it helps.

- Pick books, which interest you as it will keep your concentration better.

- With books, which are not as interesting, keep trying with them, have more breaks.

- Check with someone if you find the understanding hard.

- If you are learning something whilst reading use songs, rhymes or visual aids. In my experience if you just keep re-reading something without applying it to a picture, rhyme etc. then the brain will not retain it.

- I recently made my first ever Christmas dinner and wrote down all the instructions the night before. I took small steps and made sure I didn't get stressed. You can do this with all aspects of cooking. If you spill things, just wipe it up and keep calm. Don't worry!

- I am close to taking my driving test which has been a very big challenge for me. I have devised ways of remembering aspects of driving as my short term memory is poor. For the mirrors, I labelled each with a, b and c. I have to make sure that I look in a, then b then c mirror and it means I don't forget. When I was reversing into a parking space, I used a certain amount of bricks on the wall to help me park in the same way every time. I had to stop when I could see three bricks. Obviously you need to adapt this for the situation you are in but it can

Where's My Pen?

help. I learn best in a visual and imagining way so I wrote down on a piece of paper how to do the manoeuvres. I then imagined doing them in my head over and over again. This sounds a bit weird but it helped to process the information in my brain when I wasn't in a stressful situation of driving. The next time I practiced a parallel park, I wasn't thinking about the actual process as much but was focussing on being accurate. It worked really well for me.

- If you find directions difficult, then plan journeys whether it be on public transport or in a car. I always ask loads of people for directions, do you ever mind helping someone out who is lost? Just don't panic.

The main point to take from this chapter is to not put too much pressure on yourself. Dyspraxia or no dyspraxia, people make mistakes anyway so nobody hits perfection ever. The best thing you can do is manage your condition as calmly as you can. You are allowed days when you are frustrated but try and not let it consume you. I know it is easier said than done but try hard to take a deep breath before reacting badly to a situation. I hope you have gained something from this chapter and have started to feel more positive. Try and remember that everyone has something to offer and you can have a go at anything you want to. Just don't give up on anything.

Chapter Seven: My Tough Time and Tips on Whether to Take Medication

The following chapter will hopefully help give advice about whether taking medication is beneficial for something which occurs as a result of a LD. I am not talking about medication for dyspraxia and am not suggesting taking anti-depressants for dyspraxia. What I am doing is demonstrating the depression I went through as a result of what I believe, were dyspraxic symptoms.

My story starts when I was off from work and just not feeling myself at all, it was a surreal experience. I had an inkling that dyspraxia was causing problems but when I explained anything, it sounded wrong and I didn't explain it how it was meant to be. I said there was something wrong with my brain and the doctor thought I was saying I had a brain tumour. He/she thought I was thinking irrationally and that this was a common symptom of depression. Looking back now it was hard for the doctors as I was suggesting dyspraxia and they were saying it was just that lots of symptoms of dyspraxia were the same as symptoms for depression. I can understand this assumption but I am so upset and frustrated that no one ever said, "right, tell me how you're feeling about what you see to be dyspraxia". I feel the depression was worsened by the fact I felt trapped in my feelings of anxiety. I thought if no one was going to listen I would always find things difficult and how was I going to cope with life ever? This started my

Where's My Pen?

catastrophic thoughts and then it all spiralled into the irrational thoughts of depression. I have never been through anything quite surreal in my life. I felt like all my normal feelings and perceptions had suddenly been changed and I couldn't remember what it was like to be able to cope with everything. I don't know where the panic attacks came from and I don't know why I suddenly could not enjoy anything. If you had put a child in front of me, I would have found it hard to show love or affection towards it. That just wasn't me at all and I am now back to myself and love children and animals etc. Admittedly the depression had kicked in as a result of the stress at work and the difficulties I faced. The body has a clever way of protecting itself. I was absolutely exhausted from doing nothing and I would not wish the panic attacks on anyone.

I went from being able to cope with life to not being able to do a thing. It was like someone had come along and taken all my coping mechanisms away. This is where people do not understand depression until they have experienced it. You can't blame anyone for this as you don't know how it feels until you go through an experience. You can try and imagine what depression is like but that is coming from a sound rational mind. To actually feel like that means that you don't just feel a bit down, it totally affects your life and changes your personality. I was detached from the world, not in a deluded way but just in terms of I wasn't well. It took me so long to accept I had an illness and I felt guilty for feeling the way I did as I was lucky to have family and friends and a nice house etc. This does not matter and like any illness you cannot predict when these things may occur. It isn't a case of feeling a bit fed up it really is a change in the way the brain works whether it is chemicals etc, I do not know. The only reason I can say this now is because I am out of it: my perception of things are so different. It really wasn't a case that I could pull myself together. I remember the doctor coming around and saying I had clinical depression and I should start taking anti-depressants. It was a horrible feeling as I wanted to feel I could do it on my own. I told myself I wasn't going to take them but then when I couldn't do anything for myself and I couldn't leave the house without panicking I knew I needed help from somewhere. The issue of taking anti-depressants is so complex. I had so many opinions from family and friends, which understandably they were only trying to help. Some people said it masks the problem and others said it will just help lift me out of the worst part of depression. I guess if I am really honest I wanted someone to come along and click their fingers and I would suddenly feel a lot better. That obviously wasn't going to happen. So many people said to me, you'll get there and I never believed them. The doctor used to say, you will feel better in the future, and they just couldn't tell me when which was fair enough. They were right; it was just a long slog to the finish line.

It was really strange the first time I took the medication. I was told it may take four to six weeks to kick in and this seemed like a decade. I wasn't sure either if they were going to work. They did make me feel quite sick at first and then they made me feel really spaced out. This made me feel even worse as I was having high expectations of them helping. I think the most important piece of advice if you have to take medication is finding the correct dose and type which suits you as an individual. I went on the internet in hope that someone would say that the medication I was on was amazing and would lift me out of this awful feeling I couldn't get out of. The problem with that was, when I put the medications into google it took me to a forum where one person would say it was really good, but then someone else would say it didn't do anything and made them worse.

I really tried to persevere with the medication and I went through times when I regretted trying them. I couldn't drink alcohol with them and I really didn't feel sure about them. The doctors changed the medication to see whether any other types of anti-depressant worked. It proved to just have similar results and looking back I think they were just masking the main cause of the depression. It had become reactive depression which is depression that happens as a result of an event or something going wrong. The right medication could have helped the depression part but it would not have helped the main cause which I felt was the dyspraxia. I wasn't the type of person to just feel sorry for myself, I was always the type who tried to get on with things and be a strong person. Perhaps this is what led to the breakdown but I don't regret going through it.

The hardest part of taking the medication was that they made me so spaced out that I couldn't really function in a normal situation. When I was with my friends I felt left out of just normal things and I was so quiet. This made me paranoid that my friends would end up getting sick of me and not bother seeing me anymore. Luckily they didn't give up on me and I owe so much to them for just dragging me along with them when they went places. It wasn't easy for them granted, but they stuck by me through it all. I think they prefer the fact that they have the real me back now. You realise who your real friends are when you go through something so challenging and the people who can't handle it seem to disappear.

I was very lucky that not many people did that at all and a lot of people went out of their way to try and help me. I will never forget how much support I was given and they did genuinely keep me alive. I think the main problem with mental illness is feeling like you are on your own. I felt I was alone in the way I felt, but I was never short of support. I was very lucky and it's a shame there are people out there who do not have that support. This is where early diagnosis can prevent people suffering from depression as a result of an undiagnosed LD. I have seen it happen too much and it is such a shame. I was lucky that I came out of the depression and now am the happiest I have ever been but depression can last for years and often be hidden by people. It was amazing how many people opened up to me when I was going through the depression and admitted they knew of at least one if not more people who had been through the same thing in their life.

This is one piece of advice which I would say and that is don't give up on the medication if you find one which is not suitable. When I did find one that worked I do think it made a difference. Obviously it isn't a miracle cure but it just lifts you enough to rebuild your life again. It meant that I wasn't staying in bed all day and I could actually think a lot clearer. The problem with anti-depressants is that there can still be a stigma about them and also people do not understand the whole depression issue at times. At times, people may feel a bit down and then want to go on anti-depressants when it isn't genuine depression. This can be a bit dangerous as people can become dependent on them. I needed them but it took me a while to find the right one. I really think it is better than previous years but people still think it is a case of pulling yourself together. There are clear distinctions between being a bit down and having clinical depression. Now I am out of it I appreciate everything whether it is large or small. I really would not wish my worst enemy to go through what I felt. It was the worst part of my life although in a way it was the best thing that happened as it has totally changed my attitude to life in lots of ways.

The medication that ended up working for me was one that was combined with something else, which I can't remember the name of. Anyway, it helped me and suddenly I was able to drag myself out of my bed and into the world again. I can't tell you exactly what made me better but it's like my body shut down, it needed time out and then decided it could start all over again. I began doing voluntary work which I really enjoyed even though I was paranoid that I was too spaced out. The people were very patient with me and I also met someone who is a great friend now. The very fact that she didn't judge me for having depression made me feel that I could get better and still be involved with things. I wasn't 100% but I was getting there. I do sometimes wonder what would have happened if I hadn't taken any medication and I can't answer that. It really is a personal thing. The only thing I would say is do not feel ashamed about taking the tablets. You won't have to be on them forever and if you do then it is obviously for a reason. People do not tend to broadcast these things about being on medication so you will be surprised as to how many people are on them and you don't realise.

I haven't taken any medication for over a year now and I haven't gone back to the way I feel at all. I have had moments when I have felt down, but as mentioned before, this isn't depression; it is just feeling a bit down. There is such a massive difference and this is one thing to take from this book. I feel that a lot of mental illness is misunderstood. The problem for people going through depression, like me you don't think you will ever get out of it and this brings the despair factor. In my mind I was panicking because I didn't know what was going to happen with my life if I couldn't cope with anything. Of course this was my mind or should I say the depression playing tricks on me

Where's My Pen?

which was horrible. The positive aspect of taking medication is that it won't necessarily be forever and it is a helping hand, not a cure. It is all part of the process of making you or someone you know better. It is also a personal choice unless you are so ill you cannot make a choice for yourself. Please remember that I am not suggesting to anyone that they do take medication, it is just my experiences. It is such a personal choice. Please don't feel like you will have depression forever, there is a way out of it and there is help out there. Keep going. I used to hate people saying "you'll get there", but I did and it's great when you feel better and enjoy experiences more. Do not be afraid to contact a doctor if you are feeling really low and having any symptoms as I have described.

Chapter Eight: Alternative Therapies And Treatments

I remember one day feeling so frustrated and desperate for someone to just take me seriously that I wasn't just seeking attention for no reason. People can never feel what you're thinking, which is tough sometimes. I tried several treatments such as hypnotherapy and counselling but at the time I don't think I was ready to respond to any type of treatment.

In my research or should I say desperation, I came across a treatment called reiki. This is an energy treatment which involves working with energy channels similar to acupuncture and tai chi and providing ways of healing to humans, animals and plants. Just like people can have different opinions about LDs, it can be the same for alternative therapies. In my experience I think some people are open to trying new or alternative treatments and others will block them without even finding out if it could help them. I am open to things and find out about them, try them, and then I can be a better judge of it myself. I had an interest in reiki when I had heard about it but I didn't know anything about it. It exceeded my expectations and I now use it as a tool to help me in a lot of situations in life.

Reiki can be done on yourself and others. It is non invasive as you do not have to make contact with any part of the body if the client does not wish. You can place or hover your hands over someone whilst

Where's My Pen?

the energy goes through your body/hands to provide a healing experience. The reason I believe in it is because I feel heat and pins/needles from my hands, which I had never felt before I did the reiki courses. My teacher said to me also that levels of anxiety can reduce and the way you approach life can alter. For me this has been very true. Although obviously I feel emotions, I do not feel as panicky and anxious as I used to. It is a far cry from the panic attacks I used to have in supermarkets.

As well as being a calming influence, it can have benefits for relieving symptoms of how people are feeling. For example, I won't claim that I can cure everything, but it may relieve a headache or stomach ache and often aids sleep. People have reported to me that they have had a more relaxing sleep.

This is just one example of a therapy which has really helped me and it demonstrates that there is something out there for everyone. I have ended up becoming a master teacher in reiki so this has also given me a focus on a new skill as well as having benefit from a treatment. If you open yourself up to an opportunity you don't know where it could lead to so don't give up. At the same time I am not encouraging you to go out and spend lots of money on all treatments but there are ways around finding something which suits you. Even though therapies can be expensive, sometimes people need students to train and practice on. This can sometimes be free and you always get a supervisor who oversees the person training so it is usually safe and effective.

I feel that when you go through a tough time on a personal level and you have to really analyse your feelings and situation, it either makes you want to help others or avoid it completely. I wanted to help other people and so completed a counselling level two course. I have had both counselling and also done a course, which I found therapeutic in itself. It allows you to explore some aspects of yourself that you may not have thought about before. It also makes you appreciate the importance of empathy, i.e. putting yourself in someone else's shoes. Just from finding out about two treatments I have achieved two certificates and qualifications and also met some amazing people along the way. Therefore, when I look back I can see positive outcomes from going through a tough time.

Counselling gives you chance to vent your frustrations and just be heard. This could avoid frustration building up and then coming out in several forms like aggression. The counsellor will listen to you without making judgement and you can be yourself.

The first point of contact if you hope to get an assessment for dyspraxia, is usually through a doctor. Often through the process, they may refer you to an occupational therapist (OT) who may help with aspects like co-ordination and organisational skills. This can be very useful. Advice about how to use dyspraxic friendly equipment like tin openers and pens with appropriate grips can be really useful. I always ended losing my pen, hence the name of the book! By seeing an OT, it is not saying you can't do anything, it is just looking at practical things you may find tricky. I think I would have benefited at an early age from seeing an OT for pen control and grip help. My writing was and still is really messy so it would have been good to get support with fine motor skills (this is what we mean by things like writing, cutting for example).

Even though I have only highlighted a few therapies from this chapter, it is meant to demonstrate that you can benefit from people and treatments and you don't know where it can lead to in your life. I felt very selfish when I was going through the depression because it is almost like you're living in a bubble as you are immersed with your thoughts and situation. It wasn't intentional, but now I am well again I can give something back and hopefully people will benefit from the advice given. I feel one of the best ways of finding out about treatments is to talk to people or if that is difficult, ask someone you know to help you find out about them no matter what age you are. Good luck with everything and again, do not give up!

The next interest for me is Cognitive Behavioural Therapy (CBT), which looks at changing the way people think in order to make people feel more positive. For example, someone could think they are useless because they have a LD and give up. On the other hand, they could accept in their mind that this won't change, but there are ways to cope and manage life more effectively. If I had taken the first approach, this book would never have been published. CBT seems to be used for depression nowadays and I feel it could also be used effectively with LDs. I am interested in finding out more about it. Hopefully I will be able to help others with this therapy as well.

Where's My Pen?

Chapter Nine: For Anyone Who Knows Someone with Dyspraxia!

During my work I have spoken to many parents who feel they don't know where to get support and information about dyspraxia. This is another reason for me to write this book, in order to increase people's knowledge about the condition. It is always difficult for people to totally understand what it is like to go through something until they experience it, especially if someone hides their feelings. The first piece of advice to friends or family is not to try and assume things. It is often impossible to be psychic if someone finds it hard to explain their feelings but try and be patient and listen to what they help they feel they need.

- Be patient if someone appears scatty-they know what they want to do, but it takes a bit longer. If they are anything like me, they may put themselves down. This is linked to the frustration of finding things difficult so try and encourage them and genuinely praise what they can do. Be aware that people will most probably have a determined streak; this is a positive thing that comes out of dyspraxia. Due to the problems, we are still determined to overcome them. Even though people struggle with things they can do them, so they will achieve it. It may take them just a bit longer to process the information. It doesn't mean they are not intelligent though.

- Be aware that not many people do know what dyspraxia is so you may find yourself explaining the symptoms.

- Be patient if someone is trying to explain something as they will know what they want to say but may find it hard to formulate the order of the sentences. I used to prepare in my head exactly what I was going to say so it sounded right, but the moment had passed by the time I had done it.

- Maybe encourage people to write down their feelings. It doesn't matter if they find it hard as they may find it easier to write than speak (just depends on the person).

- Realise that household chores may be tricky e.g. the order of cleaning a bathroom or cooking. I always wanted to do everything at once even though I was aware it should be done in a certain order.

- Try and imagine a situation where you find something difficult. Everyone finds something difficult, but can often learn how to overcome it.

- People with dyspraxia may be aware of their problem but may need help to overcome it. For example, I am aware of everything I find hard, but not always sure how to go about correcting in myself.

Where's My Pen?

- Try and encourage an individual to face a problem but in a controlled environment. I am not saying if they don't like heights to jump out of a plane, but if they find travelling independently hard then go with them gradually and then let them do small steps by themselves. Give constant reassurance that they shouldn't avoid the things they don't feel comfortable with. There are ways around this. The example I have used somewhere in this book involved me facing my fear of answering the phone. It did really help me when I answered the phone non-stop for a while. Perhaps this won't work for everyone, but there are ways of adapting activities to overcome challenges. Just give it a go and see what happens!

- Try and educate friends and family about the symptoms of dyspraxia. I have spoken to members of a family whose grandson has dyspraxia and they said "I'm really worried that he doesn't keep his room tidy and he sits there staring at the mess and not knowing how to tidy up". She didn't realise this can be a symptom of dyspraxia and individuals can find it hard to organise themselves. It doesn't have to be overwhelming like you're preaching about the condition; just let them know the basics. See the leaflet you can print out and give to others.

- Perhaps try and ask the person with dyspraxia, what support they think they need? Often others can think they know the right approach where the actual person isn't consulted about anything.

As long as the person feels supported I think this makes such a difference. I think if a person feels positive they will thrive more in a situation. It is basic psychology that a negative environment will not be conducive to raising self esteem compared to a positive and supportive situation. For example, if you say "I can't believe you can't tie your laces, you're a nightmare!", then obviously this will not have any benefit to developing self esteem. On the other hand, if you say "right, I know you will be able to tie your laces so we'll work on it in stages", then this allows someone to think they can achieve it and they have the support at the same time.

I really hope you will take something from these tips even if it is just one piece of advice. If you feel strongly about supporting people with dyspraxia why not start a support group so people can talk about their experiences. There are opportunities out there to be taken so give it a go!

Where's My Pen?

Chapter Ten: Dyspraxia and Posture

The following chapter looks at physical aspects of having dyspraxia and ways which could help to prevent further problems occurring in later life.

You could imagine dyspraxia being that the mind knows what the body wants to do but it doesn't always do this. Therefore, it can appear that a body is clumsy and out of control just because the brain finds it hard to correct movements quickly. This means that often muscles can appear quite weak and floppy. It is not necessarily that the muscles are weak; it could be that it is the lack of control over the muscles which make the posture appear floppy or tense. For example, my friends always used to tell me off for my shoulders being so rounded and this was perhaps the lack of control over sitting up straight and with an upright posture. I think we are all guilty of that over-relaxed posture where we don't think about sitting up straight. However, there is a difference between someone just appearing to have floppy muscles because they can't be bothered to sit up straight and a person who has weak and floppy muscles because it is hard for them to maintain the muscle control for long periods of time.

The problem with postural differences is that they can often cause injuries to other parts of the body. For example if you have a weak back or core, i.e. the deep muscles around the middle of your body, then it can affect your knees or ankles. The core of the body is often forgotten about as it involves quite deep muscles called transverses abdominus and multifidus. I won't go into extreme detail regarding this because again, I don't want to make it too confusing. However, an important thing to think of is that these deep muscles help maintain our posture and if they are used in the correct way then they can help prevent problems with the back. It can take a while to learn how to switch these muscles on but this is where Pilates can be very useful. Beginners sessions will help you learn how to switch the muscles on and at the same time still breathe. It can often be tricky to start with but with practice it can get a lot easier. Getting a DVD to do at home could be a start if you feel more comfortable doing this.

An example of weak core stability was when I decided to try a half marathon. I always knew my posture was really bad but didn't think it would affect my running. I was looking forward to the half marathon after weeks of training really hard. At the beginning of the race, I suddenly felt like someone was hitting my knee with a hammer. It was very bizarre as it was such a new feeling to me. Admittedly I should have dropped out of the race but my determination took over and the fact I was raising money for a charity kept me going. When I got someone to look at my knee they said nothing was wrong with the knee joint but my posture was really bad so I was putting pressure on my joints. My joints are hyper mobile, which means they move a lot so can become unstable if the muscles are weak around them. Hyper means more and so

Where's My Pen?

it means more mobility, i.e. movement. As a result this meant I was injuring my knee. It may not be that all muscles are weak, but certain muscles like back muscles may cause problems if not used effectively. Exercises can be done to correct this. Although I am qualified as a physiotherapist it is advisable to consult either a doctor where they could refer you to a physiotherapist or book directly to see a private physiotherapist.

I remember when I was training we had to identify aspects of each other's posture to then imagine analysing a patient's posture. At first it seemed like mine was fine, but then when the lecturer looked more closely they realised it wasn't great. The following aspects make up my unusual posture. My feet roll inwards which can be called over-pronation and I have flat feet. Some people have higher arches in their feet than others. I don't really have any arches because my muscles are quite floppy and that could be why my feet roll inwards. Also my pelvis tilts the wrong way sometimes because my muscles are quite weak and when tired just make my pelvis drop forward instead of keeping me upright. This means that it may be a good idea if I was more aware of my posture and stood up straighter. Also I go swimming and do exercises in the gym which help. Please consult a doctor before you decide on any exercises or seek some advice to get the most appropriate exercises for your individual posture. Often people with dyspraxia may have some of the same postural differences as me. Others may not-again I am not claiming to be an expert on the matter although I am interested in this area.

I always knew my posture was awful and when trying to sit up; my body would fight against it and ache. Now I realise it is something to do with having low tone. I mentioned earlier that some people can appear to have weak and floppy muscles (scientific terms I do not think!). This could be due to low muscle tone.

In layman's terms, if muscles have a high tone there could be a lot of tension in the muscle and it is difficult to move them easily. However, if a muscle has low tone, then there could be lots of movement and not too much tension like the muscles around my back.

People with LDs may have double jointed arms and/or legs and also may have an arched back. This could point towards low tone so it may be useful to visit the GP for advice.

If someone you know with dyspraxia fidgets a lot then this could be because it is harder for someone with dyspraxia to hold their muscles in a certain position and so they will move around a lot and fidget. It takes more time for the brain to control posture because it requires a lot of motor planning, i.e. telling the brain to either execute a movement or hold a body still. I was always and still am very fidgety. Due to the hyper mobility and/or low tone, I am always sitting crossed legged and find this really comfortable. I used to get told not to sit on

Where's My Pen?

the floor but sit on a chair-but the floor was always more comfortable as I could spread out more.

Here are a few tips for helping improve your posture:

- Using a gym ball might be beneficial as this works on core stability. You could either buy a video/DVD or sit in front of the television on the ball. This will help posture as you are using muscles to keep you upright on an unstable surface i.e. the ball.

- I have tried yoga and Pilates which have both been of benefit to me. Yoga works more on the flexibility whereas Pilates focuses on core stability.

- Try going to a running shop who can give advice on footwear which may help your posture. Sometimes they will watch you run and assess which trainers you may need.

- It is more tiring for someone with dyspraxia to hold their body position as they do not have as much muscle tone. Try not to confuse this with toning your muscles up when exercising in a gym, it is different from that.

One thing that made sense to me also was when someone said the reason I never feel full after eating is because of the low tone in the stomach. If the muscles do not hold the body up in a postural sense the stomach could also be quite floppy. This is now my excuse for eating lots! At times, people with dyspraxia could potentially be overweight for this reason. Exercises would be beneficial for not only posture but keeping weight steady as well.

I am aware whilst writing this that people may question my knowledge and expertise in this area. I am qualified as a physiotherapist but I do not claim to know everything-it is merely to help with understanding of the link between posture and LDs. I would always advise a trip to a practitioner for a full assessment and appropriate advice on treatment for each individual. Treatments do not have to be a chore and often physiotherapists will devise fun activities to help children improve spatial awareness, posture and muscle strength to name a few.

Where's My Pen?

Chapter Eleven: Advantages of Being Dyspraxic

Although I'm telling everyone about all aspects of dyspraxia, there are definitely positive attributes and everyone has them even if you do not believe it!

- Because I am so aware of my poor organisational skills, I can often be more organised than others because it makes me more stressed otherwise. This has come from years of panicking because I was so scatty and disorganised. In my current work, I plan a lot of what I do, well in advance because it makes me more relaxed. The plans may change but at least I have an outline of what I am going to do.

- I may leave extra time to travel if I'm having a good day just because I hate being late. All these things just make me more determined to achieve and work hard. People with dyspraxia can be good problem solvers!

- I live by lists and the sense of achievement when you tick them off feels good. It helps to organise the day and week for example.

- From this extra effort put in, it makes a person more appealing to an employer and this is positive. A lot of people I have met with dyspraxia are very hard workers. If you are reading this thinking someone with dyspraxia is lazy, it could just be because they tire more easily than others.

- Majority of individuals with dyspraxia may have a good sense of humour, which often is used as a cover up or coping mechanism. However, it is good to have this quality. I think when I started to put less pressure on myself and laugh more; I started to feel more relaxed. No one can do everything all of the time and often people feel anxious about things but appear confident. Maybe the frustration can kick in for a short while because this is only a natural reaction, but the most important thing is to be able to laugh at yourself and with others. It doesn't have to always end in frustration and anger. This isn't to say we will not feel like that from time to time but I think a lot of people with dyspraxia have an inner strength, which is definitely a positive attribute.

- People do not give up and although get frustrated, are determined to achieve something.

- A lot of children and adults with a LD have achieved a lot of amazing things in their lives and I have a lot of admiration for them. I think even if something is hard, people will try hard and use determination to pull them through. This could often be mistaken for stubbornness but either way, determination can definitely be another positive characteristic. If you take some

Where's My Pen?

famous people with LDs they have achieved amazing results. One task for you is to research in whatever way suits you and find out if there are any famous people with dyspraxia. You may be surprised at what names come up.

- A lot of people are big fans of children and animals and will have a very caring and empathic side.

Again, I am not saying that everyone who has dyspraxia will love children and animals but this could be a positive attribute. I am naturally drawn to children and animals and always have been. Maybe it is because my caring side does not require technical ability and co-ordination, it requires love and patience. That sounds a bit corny but it is true. I am very patient with people and have a lot of empathy and often people with LDs are very empathic.

- People may be patient with others because they know what it is like to find things tricky.

I have mentioned this briefly before but once people with dyspraxia do understand an instruction, often they are very able and excel at what they are doing. This is an exception with me and skiing but we can't have everything in life! Sometimes it may just take a bit longer to process instructions but it may mean that people consider safety more because they may be afraid of making a mistake. I do voluntary work which involves first aid and so I make sure that I don't put anyone in danger. I have probably read more about first aid than maybe others because of this reason. I ask lots of questions which may annoy a lot of people but if it avoids a dangerous situation then it is better to ask. It shows your brain is still working and not just following others.

There are often different types of intelligence and people in general may excel in one thing but find something else really difficult. It is important to remember this so you don't put too much pressure on yourself when you're feeling down or frustrated.

The main positive aspect of dyspraxia is that anything is possible. There is always a way around things so do not give up! Stay positive.

Where's My Pen?

Chapter Twelve: Dyspraxia in the Workplace

If you carried out research on people such as prisoners and the unemployed, I could imagine that at least a few individuals have a LD which has gone unnoticed. If they are not recognised, a lot of individuals may think they cannot achieve anything and feel they might as well be caught up in crime. If they haven't had the attention they need to find something to suit their skills, they are often forgotten. I think this is very sad and another reason for trying to diagnose children/adults at an early age. This motivates me to keep writing this book.

During work I have come across different perceptions of LDs, some very supportive, others not sympathetic at all. I think the first main important thing to think of as obvious as it sounds is that people will always react in different ways; that accounts for lots of aspects of life. One person will understand your symptoms and may help you in the utmost way; others may not understand the condition and will be impatient. The important thing is to try and rationalise this and not take things too personally. Again, it is sometimes easier said than done but have a go. I have had people tell me that, no you can't be dyspraxic; you did two degrees, blah blah blah. I feel like saying, "oh of course, I thought I would just make it up for fun and ask for sympathy". Coping strategies and cover–ups have a funny way of hiding things.

I still struggle at work sometimes as I never know when to ask for more help. A few times I have thought, oh I could do with extra time for that but then felt I was being a pain and didn't want to bother anyone. This is probably one of the worst things to do as if you end up making a mistake and it comes back on you. Your employer will then wonder why didn't ask for help. Try not to let pride stand in the way and just ask for help. You may realise that lots of people are struggling as well but not making it apparent. In my present job, I have been offered extra support which means a lot to me and it makes me more motivated to do a good job. Personally for me, if someone does not understand then it is really challenging for me. For the first time I really feel like someone is listening to me and that really makes a difference. I now have a job where I support people who have a disability and I empathise and really try and see it from their perspective. I try and listen to what they want, not what I think they should be doing.

Here are a few tips on coping with getting a job:

Researching for the job:

If you prefer, perhaps you can find out if certain companies are more supportive towards people with LDs. Every employer should make suitable adjustments for any individual who has a disability. The Disability Discrimination Act 1995, states that an employer should legally make reasonable adjustments at work for someone with a disability. There is no reason why somebody with dyspraxia should not be able to carry out a job in a positive way. Ultimately you also have to make the decision as to whether to tell them about the condition. I believe that if an employer is worth working for you should be able to tell them without them passing specific judgement. Obviously this will make them think in a slightly different way but they would have to in order to help you. However, what they don't realise is that by having a slightly different way of thinking you can often think laterally and come up with solutions which others would not think of. Therefore, remember you can be a benefit to the company. When researching the job, if you need help with filling in forms and understanding jargon don't be afraid to ask. Again, others will also find aspects of forms hard to decipher.

Here is an example of two ways to approach an interview or writing on an application form:

Example A:

I have dyspraxia so I won't be very good at some things; I find quite a lot of things hard to do so think I will be rubbish.

Example B:

I have dyspraxia so there may be some areas of my work I may need support with. However, I am very willing to try my hardest and it will not stop me from doing a good job.

Example B would be the best one to use as it is positive and if somebody reads the first example it portrays negative feelings about the dyspraxia and yourself.

Preparing for the interview:

I always prepared things that I wanted to say in the interview before-hand. Obviously you don't know exactly what they will ask but it is better to write some aspects of yourself down, in case they ask the usual questions like "what are your strengths and weaknesses?"

You can research your employment rights before you go to an interview and you can have someone to support you if you need it.

For my recent job interview, I mentioned that I have a personal experience of a LD and I felt this would be positive to support others in a similar situation. When I got the job, I then explained more about dyspraxia and my individual situation which helped the employer understand more about me.

You could say, "I sometimes find certain things difficult due to dyspraxia but it is also an advantage because of ..... and I feel I have been able to achieve things so far and it makes me more determined to get the best out of the job I do". As long as it doesn't come across as negative, they will respect you for being honest and trying to achieve something for yourself.

Where's My Pen?

Prepare your smart clothes the night before and perhaps do a practice run to the interview because you may find directions difficult. This will make you feel more relaxed before your interview.

If you get the job, sorry when you get the job!!

When you get the job, congratulate yourself because you have done well and achieved that job you went for. Now, if you haven't already disclosed dyspraxia then you can either be honest with your manager if they seem approachable or not say anything. There is no right or wrong approach, it is just how much you want to disclose to people. At least if you say something the employer is aware of your feelings and support you may need. Consider the following aspects of the work environment:

- Postural awareness, e.g. are the chairs supportive to your back if you are sitting for long periods of time?

- Do you need extra time or support for reading documents or preparing for something if understanding is required?

- Do you understand what the role entails and are there areas which you could prepare for before you start your job?

- By checking with your manager if there is anything you could read etc. This is showing initiative and can be helpful for you too.

- Try and get as many details about starting times, rotas, lunchtimes etc.

- Try and get a comfortable uniform or clothes to work in so you are comfy in your work and not worrying. By eliminating all the little stressful bits it can make you feel less nervous about starting work.

- Best of all, enjoy it! Don't put too much pressure on yourself in the first week-you are new to everything. Learn things in small chunks, take a notebook if need be. It could be a funky colourful one and again it is showing initiative.

Overall, do not be afraid to apply for jobs. You can apply for benefits through the jobcentre if you have a disability, but just think how positive it would be to go into the world of work and meet new people! There is no reason why you cannot use your positive skills and attributes. Just go for it! Good luck.

Where's My Pen?

Chapter Thirteen: A Future with Dyspraxia

I've learnt over the years that in lots of different situations there will always be a way to solve a problem. This keeps me positive. It may not always be the preferred choice or the nicest choice but there is always a way. Since adopting this attitude I'm less prone to panicking and more likely to take a deep breath, think about the situation and adapt to the situation accordingly. For example. Situation 1:

You spill a drink over someone in front of you in front of everyone.

Solution 1:

You panic, try to run and get a cloth , panic more as you don't know where to get from and trip over your feet. It ends with you getting frustrated and upset and then maybe crying.

Solution 2:

Go oops, laugh and take a deep breath. Calmly get up, someone may have already come with a cloth or if not, go and ask the bar person if in a pub or café. They will advise you accordingly. Try and rationalise the situation and say to yourself that no one was hurt (hopefully not) and pride may have been dented a wee bit but still intact. A counsellor once went through a process with me that didn't help me at the time but now it makes complete sense. She takes the situation and says, "right you've spilt a drink, what's the worst that can happen?" I answer, "I feel stupid" and she says, "yes but what is the worst that can happen". She keeps going on like this and in the end you realise that nothing is going to happen. I realise that bad things do happen in the world but what I'm trying to say is that often in a lot of situations are not as bad as you may think they are. I have to be honest and say I am not superhuman so cannot adopt this theory 100% all the time but it does seem to help in lots of situations in my life and gives me more confidence to have a go at different activities.

Just because you find some things hard to do and learn, it also means you have valuable skills to offer. I tend to think in different ways so can often come up with solutions that others may not have thought of. Remember what the supportive people say and forget what the other, negative, unsupportive people say. In lots of different issues in life you will come across people who challenge what you feel strongly about and may upset you a lot. Try and stick with what you believe in and don't get upset.

Chapter Fourteen: Finding A Diagnosis, Should I Be Labelled?

There are different perceptions about whether someone should get a diagnosis for anything these days. Some people feel being labelled is a negative perception and others feel it is positive as they know why they feel the way they do. I would feel better if someone said to me, "yes you are dyspraxic", as I really wondered what was wrong with me when I was younger. I spent far too long feeling inferior to my peers and not enough time enjoying life. I have made up for it already and would not have written this book otherwise. For me, the best thoughts to have are that it is personal to every individual. I feel it can often be people who know nothing about LDs who pass the judgement. If you ask some people, who are making negative comments, if they know anything about LDs, often they don't or they have wrong information. This I guess is a form of ignorance, hence another reason for writing this book. People I have spoken to have found it hard to decide whether to get a diagnosis. I guess after all is said and done, you are who you are. However, it has made a massive difference beyond belief for me to focus on something which may be a reason for my difficulties.

If after reading this book, you are thinking that either you or someone you know may have dyspraxia, then you could do the following:

- Contact the doctor.

- Be aware that not all doctors may know what the condition is. Try and give them a book like this to read.

- Be persistent as they may have waiting lists for assessment and be reluctant to do anything.

- Try and write down symptoms and let them know you have researched the condition.

- What may happen is that the doctor may refer you to an educational or general psychologist for an assessment. They can often give a diagnosis.

- You can go private and pay for a psychologist but this can be pricey.

Just remember you do not have to do anything if you feel happy to carry on as you are. On the contrary, if you think you would like to but do not know how to do it, then contact the doctor. Take someone with you and this doesn't matter how young or old you are.

For parents who are wondering whether to tell their children about a diagnosis which already may have been given, again, it is very individual. I worked with someone who was very young but very articulate about having Asperger Syndrome and I felt respect for him for being so open. This could help him make others feel proud of their positive

Where's My Pen?

skills and strengths. It depends what the diagnosis means to a person. As said earlier, some people may draw strength from it and try and support others with LDs.

The positive aspect of being diagnosed with a LD suggests that you are of either average or above average intelligence. This means that peoples' brains just work in a different way but this can be a positive thing.

Don't be afraid to seek help from charities or organisations. You will be amazed at how you can find things out just by talking to people about the condition. They may know people who work in the field or who suffer from it. Good luck and do not give up if you feel you want a diagnosis.

For children, if they receive a diagnosis, they may get statemented at school. This means they are entitled to get extra help in school for work they may struggle with. Speak to a teacher about this if you want more information. There tends to be more special needs co-ordinators now so hopefully the teacher or the doctor can help.

I hope this has been informative and the main piece of advice is keep asking for help whether it be in school, talking to the doctor, or in the work environment. You are not superhuman!

Chapter Fifteen: S.O.S. To A Bad Dyspraxic Day

This was written before I was made redundant and used to work with both children and adults with LDs.

Cor blimey, if I bump into anything else today then I will cry! I start the day feeling like I am dropping everything and even before I get to work; I win the award for running up and down the stairs the most as I keep forgetting things for work, like pens, keys, money, and the list goes on! I make mistakes that are so silly and feel like the world is spiralling out of control around me. Well, ok a slight exaggeration but it's not a fun day for me. Thankfully there are always children at work with words of wisdom to cheer me up when I am feeling sorry for myself. I would say 80% of the time I laugh things off and make a joke but the odd times the frustration builds and I have a little cry. I know this may seem like a weakness but I think it's my body just having time out. I feel a lot better for it that's for sure. There are those times where you want to crawl into that hidden hole where no one can see all your mistakes you are making. For me it's the days when it seems like I am walking around with a big sign on my head saying 'I am having a rubbish day' (to put it politely!) Okay, so how do you handle it? I'm always better at giving out the advice as opposed to taking it so here goes:

Where's My Pen?

- Try hard to accept that some days are worse than others especially if tiredness creeps in.

- Try and channel your frustration, either with deep breaths or getting fresh air. Today I walked around the block and it made such a difference. It's the simple things that at times are the best remedy.

- Try and empathise with someone else because if you channel your energies to something or someone else then it is taking your mind off your own problems.

- Write lists constantly for the whole day to take the emphasis off having to remember things causing you more stress.

- Remember that it will pass and you will have a better day soon. Try and laugh it off or make a joke. My friend's dad said you don't have to be miserable to be serious and I think that's right.

- Try hard to think of your good points (although it is hard if you feel frustrated and annoyed).

- Have a good sing song to your favourite music and dance around like there is no-one watching!

- Try and do an activity like yoga or tai chi to relax you.

- Talk to people who know about your problems. They should understand and if they don't then go to someone else who does.

- Try not to dwell for too long, make it more productive so at least you can do something. After all, the world won't end if you drop a cup and trip over your dog!

Where's My Pen?

Chapter Sixteen: Life Nowadays and General Feeling about Learning Difficulties

Well, I can safely say that my life is the best it has ever been although my dyspraxia isn't cured. I don't think it will ever totally go away but I have learnt from it in so many ways. What's the difference now? I don't take myself too seriously. Doesn't mean to say I don't get down about things, I am only human. However, I am now not bothered if I trip up in public. If I make a fool of myself, what is the worst that happens? I go red; get a bit embarrassed then what happens-absolutely nothing. Obviously things can happen but a lot of the time they are out of our hands. It is better to have a go rather than wishing you had tried something. Now be realistic as well. I'm not suggesting you do a parachute jump without a parachute (you get my drift don't you!). Just laugh, this is what I have learnt. When you take the pressure off yourself, people warm to you more and enjoy your company more. Don't worry if you genuinely get upset and have to cry, that's alright. However just try and rationalise things. Again, I know it is easier said than done, but try and put things into perspective.

I work with adults with LDs and empathy I think is a big thing. If someone knows that you have been through something similar it does go a long way. Believe me; people who had gone through depression were very supportive because of their own experiences.

During 2008 I was made redundant as the company had to close, but it has also taught me that you can get through anything and it can often turn out better in the end. I am really happy now and have enjoyed writing this book. Even though sometimes it has been hard to put ideas down from head to paper, it has still been a big achievement for me and will always remember this experience.

Because I have been at my lowest, I can now feel my best as every day I know I want to get out of bed and make the most out of my day. I have achieved so many things in the past few years and it has made me realise you can have a go at things, enjoy them and succeed in them. If you think in a negative way, it will probably result in a negative result. Keep trying your best and that is all you can do at any age. Keep going and good luck. You can do it!

Where's My Pen?

My General Feeling about Learning Difficulties

The more and more people I talk to the more I realise that something needs to be done to raise awareness about LDs. People, who are not knowledgeable about LDs, may take the wrong approach towards someone with a LD. The work I am doing at the moment involves people with autism. Now there are many types of symptoms and people who are on different scales of the autistic spectrum. Therefore, one person with autism could be quite different to another. The problem is that people may place individuals into similar categories even when they are different. Assumptions can be made and when it comes to creating a future for people, conclusions can be jumped to and skills are often overlooked. I have mentioned it a few times during this book but I really feel strongly that people should know more about these conditions. It surely wouldn't come as such a surprise as well if you had a child with one of these conditions. People can live happy lives and I know several people with LDs who are very intelligent and have achieved high marks in their studies. It is really hard because with a physical disability you can see what is wrong; with a LD it cannot always be seen. Also, if someone is in public and acts a bit differently or has challenging behaviour, often people will not know the reason for it. If awareness was better, perhaps people would be more patient with others.

Since working with Aspergers and autism, it has made me realise that throughout the whole spectrum of LDs I often feel self esteem is knocked by other people who do not understand these conditions. I have had some corkers of comments said to me like, "you don't look as though you've got a disability". It isn't necessarily anyone's fault if they don't know anything about these conditions, but it surely isn't difficult to teach them at school either. Surely information about LDs could be added into the curriculum somewhere? I have had some really interesting conversations with people about dyspraxia and I feel there are a lot of people who would want to know more about learning difficulties/disabilities/differences.

Here are some general words of advice for anyone with any LD:

- Never feel it is your problem that you have a LD, try and explain to someone who doesn't know about it.

- Don't give up, there may be times when you feel low in confidence, but you can do it. Keep going!!

- Don't be embarrassed about asking for help. If you achieve something well because you asked one question then what's the harm in that. You are showing initiative and this is positive.

Where's My Pen?

- Think of at least one goal you want to achieve and make sure you do it or do it with help. Remember how it makes you feel when you've achieved it.

- Try and find out about other LDs as sometimes people can get wrapped up in their own challenges.

- Try and keep your life as organised as you can so you don't feel more anxious.

- People are only trying to help if they suggest something, do not be stubborn about it! (talking from personal experience!).

- Take life in small steps, one step at a time, so you don't feel anxious about something in the future. This will go a long way to achieving success.

I hope to achieve a lot more in my life and hope people reading this will contact me and let me know if it has helped in any way. I have worked with some very special people, both children and adults. If you are reading this and I have worked with you, I really hope you will go for what you want to achieve and what you believe in. Keep positive and do not give up. Thank you for taking the time to read this book and hope you've got to the end and enjoyed everything you have read.

References and Useful Contacts

I mentioned somewhere in the book that I didn't want to review lots of literature because I wanted it to be a down to earth guide. However, I have to reference the information I took from the definitions of dyspraxia and there are a few useful websites which I hope is helpful to you all. I'm sure you will find your own so good luck!

1) www.dyspraxiafoundation.org.uk

For further advice and support for dyspraxia

2) En.wikipedia.org

   Used for a definition of 'dys' and 'praxis'.

3) www.jobcentreplus.gov.uk

   www.direct.gov.uk

   For advice regarding disability rights

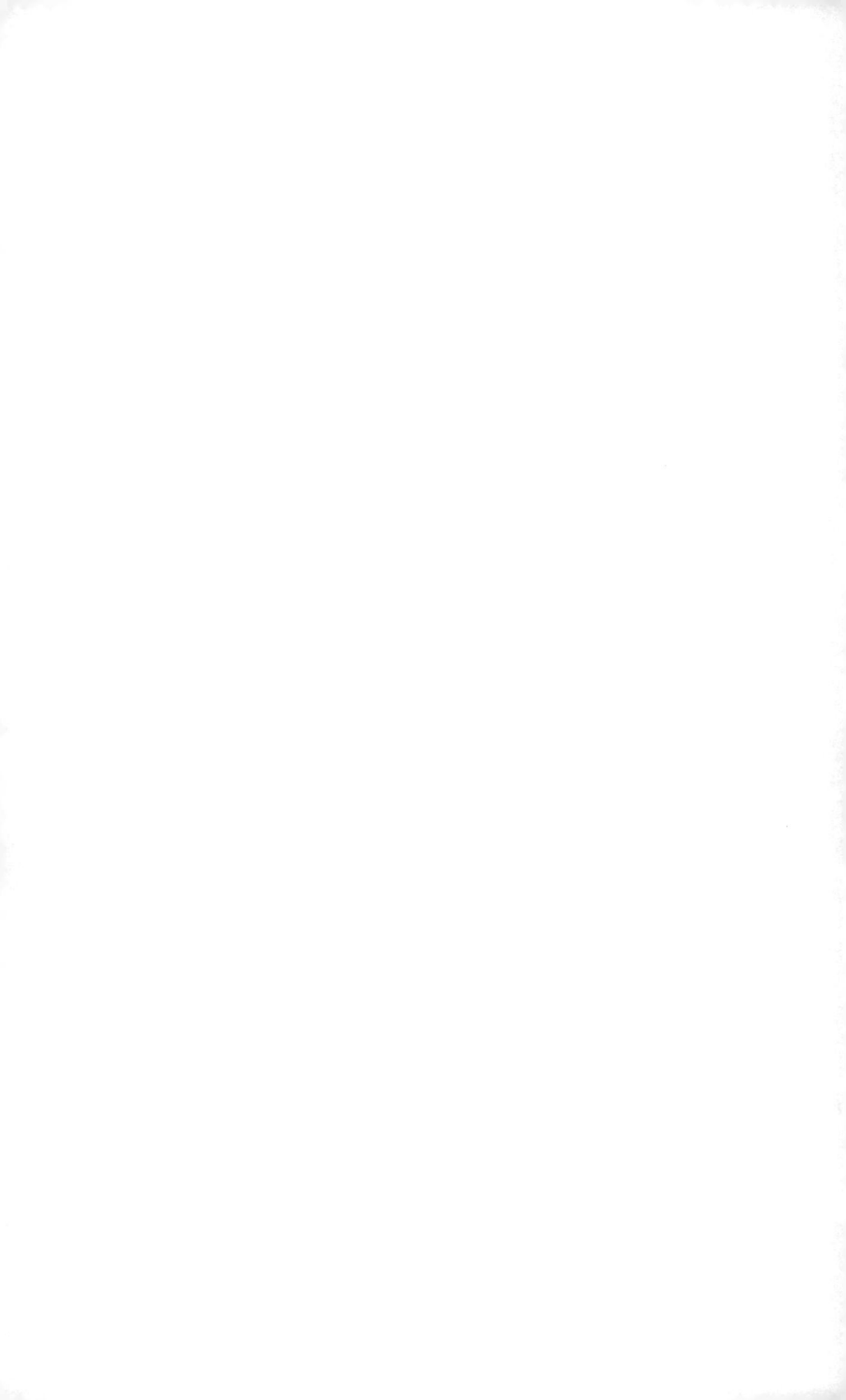

www.ingramcontent.com/pod-product-compliance
Ingram Content Group UK Ltd.
Pitfield, Milton Keynes, MK11 3LW, UK
UKHW041412180426
11947UKWH00007B/78